OBESITY

Dr. Girish Gadkari

Elaine Coveney

MERCURY LEARNING AND INFORMATION

Dulles, Virginia | Boston, Massachusetts | New Delhi

Publisher: David Pallai
MERCURY LEARNING AND INFORMATION
22841 Quicksilver Drive
Dulles, VA 20166
info@merclearning.com
www.merclearning.com
1-800-758-3756

This book is printed on acid-free paper.

Dr. Girish Gadkari and Elaine Coveney. *Obesity.*
ISBN: 978-1-937585-86-0

Library of Congress Control Number: 2012956349

1314321

Printed in the United States of America

Our titles are available for adoption, license, or bulk purchase by
associations, universities, corporations, etc.
For additional information, please contact the Customer Service Dept. at
1-800-758-3756 (toll free) or info@merclearning.com.

Contents

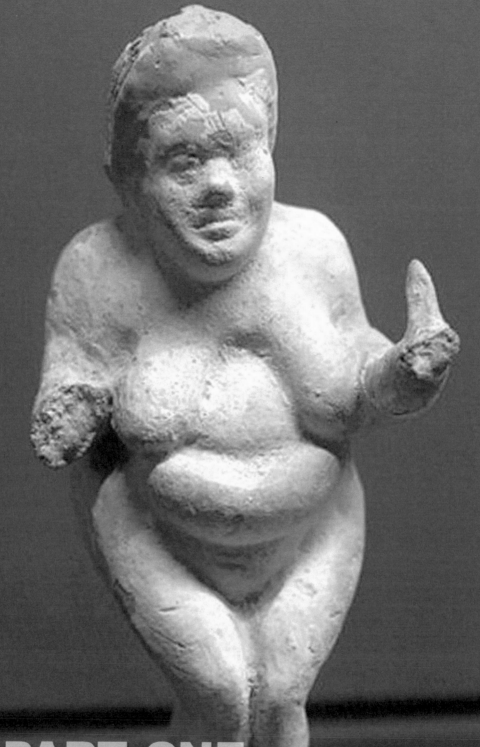

PART ONE

Obesity Basics

In Part One, we define what obesity is and show you how to calculate your BMI (body mass index), probably the most used gauge of obesity. We also cover the limitations of BMI as an obesity measure, talk about other methods of assessing your body-fat percentage, and tell you which kind of fat is most dangerous to your health. We then outline the causes, prevalence, and contributing factors for obesity. A discussion of obesity in children and adolescents follows, including factors that are specific to the development of obesity in young people and its physiological and psychological impacts on them. Finally, we examine the health risks associated with obesity.

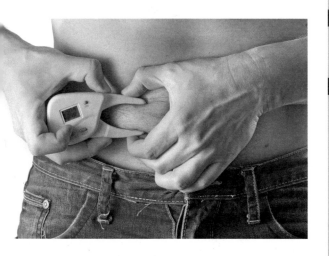

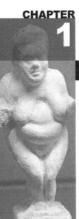

CHAPTER 1 *Obesity and Its Causes*

1. What is obesity?

In the United States alone over two-thirds of adults and almost 49 percent of young people ages 2–19 are considered either obese or overweight, and rates are at alarming levels around the world as well.[1] The speed at which this has happened makes it clear that it is no overstatement to speak of the "obesity epidemic."

> **Obesity** can be defined as excess weight compared to the height of an individual, but the term specifically applies to individuals with an excess of **adipose tissue** (fat). People who are 10–20 percent above normal weight (according to a standard weight-and-height chart) are usually classified as overweight, while those who are 20 percent or more above normal weight are usually classified as obese. These thresholds help medical professionals identify people who carry too much fat, but not all individuals who fall within these parameters are overweight or obese.
>
> **DEFINITION**

For an overview of what's caused the obesity epidemic and what we need to do to bring obesity rates down, see Video1.1.Epidemic.

ON THE DVD

Excessive weight is associated with a number of serious health conditions—among them diabetes and heart disease—that increase the risk for premature death. The high costs of obesity in particular to human well-being and global medical systems make reducing its prevalence one of the most important health challenges of our time.

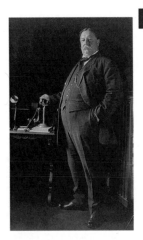

2. How can I tell if I'm obese?

Currently, **body mass index (BMI)** is the measure used most often to determine whether an individual is obese. BMI is defined as an individual's body mass (weight) in kilograms, divided by his or her height in meters squared. A conversion factor is used to calculate BMI if pounds and inches, or pounds and feet, are used.

BMI charts generally classify weight-to-height ratios into four categories (see Table 1.1), and thresholds for the *overweight* and *obese* categories have been set at different levels over the years. The ones currently in use in the United States were adopted from the World Health Organization (WHO) in 1998.

TABLE 1.1 BMI weight categories

BMI	WEIGHT STATUS
< 18.50	Underweight
18.50–24.99	Normal
25–29.99	Overweight
30 and above	Obese

SOURCE: World Health Organization, Global Database on Body Mass Index, http://apps.who.int/bmi/index.jsp?introPage=intro_3.html

The *obese* category is subdivided into three groups:
* Class I, BMI 30–34.99 (moderately obese)
* Class II, BMI 35–39.99 (severely obese)
* Class III, BMI 40 and above (very severely or morbidly obese)

3. How is BMI calculated?

For adults, BMI is calculated as follows:
* Multiply your weight (in pounds) by 703
* Divide that number by your height (in inches)
* Divide that number by your height again

For example, if you're 5 feet 4 inches tall (64 inches) and weigh 150 pounds, your BMI would be:

* 150 × 703 = 105,450
* 105,450 / 64 = 1647.66
* 1647.66 / 64 = 25.74

A BMI of 25.74 would place you in the overweight category on the chart shown in Table 1.1.

Keep in mind that BMI is a proxy for estimating an individual's percentage of body fat and does not always accurately reflect how much fat a person carries. One limitation

The method for determining BMI for children is different from the method used for adults and is discussed in Question 9.

For a BMI calculator, visit:

http://www.cdc.gov/healthyweight/assessing/bmi/index.html

or

http://www.crestor.com/c/your-arteries/tools-resources/bmi-calculator.aspx

To determine your body frame size, visit:

http://www.livestrong.com/article/169271-how-to-determine-body-frame/

ON THE WEB

is that BMI does not take **body frame** (skeleton) size into account—the larger the frame, the higher the ideal weight range applicable to an individual.

A second problem with BMI as a measure of body fat is that people who are fit or athletic can end up in the *overweight* or *obese* categories in BMI charts because of their higher muscle mass.

BMI can also provide a distorted picture of fat levels in very short and very tall individuals, and can underestimate the amount of body fat in people who are older or who have lost muscle. Moreover, BMI thresholds apply to both men and women, even though women carry about 10 percent more fat than men for any given BMI value. BMI, therefore, may underestimate obesity in women.

Finally, a serious limitation of BMI is that it says nothing about the distribution of body fat, which is important in evaluating risk levels for health problems associated with obesity (such as heart attacks).

4. Is BMI the only way to tell how much body fat I have?

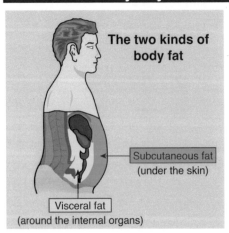

The two kinds of body fat

Subcutaneous fat (under the skin)

Visceral fat (around the internal organs)

There are different terms for the fat in your body (see Figure 1.1):

Subcutaneous fat lies just under the skin.

Visceral fat is located in the abdominal cavity between and around the organs.

Abdominal (belly) fat consists of both visceral and subcutaneous fat.

◀ FIGURE 1.1
Subcutaneous versus visceral fat.

The location of adipose tissue has important implications for your health. Subcutaneous fat in the thighs and buttocks, for example, is much less dangerous than any kind of belly fat.

Probably the simplest way to determine the amount of abdominal fat you have—the fat associated with higher risks of heart and other diseases (see Chapter 3)—is to measure your **waist circumference**. Determining your **waist-to-hip ratio** will give you an even better idea of how much belly fat you have. (To calculate the ratio, simply divide the circumference of your waist by the circumference of your hips.)

ON THE WEB

For a rundown on different kinds of fat, visit:

http://www.webmd.com/diet/features/the-truth-about-fat

ON THE WEB

For guidelines on how to measure yourself correctly, as well as tables that predict risk to cardiovascular health based on your results, visit:

http://www.youtube.com/watch?v=jyL8UfGZMJE

Body-fat monitors and **body-fat scales** for home use are now widely available. Both use **bioelectrical impedance analysis (BIA)**—wherein a light, harmless electrical current passes through the body—to assess body fat. BIA acts on the principle that lean tissue conducts more current because it is composed of more water than fat (about 75 percent versus about 10 percent). Devices record the amount of current that is repelled and conducted; the percentage repelled is your estimated body-fat percentage. Because measurements depend on water content in the body, which can be fairly variable, results also can be variable.

Calipers can be used to measure **skinfold thickness** at different sites (see Figure 1.2); measurements are then fed into an equation to figure out the percentage of subcutaneous fat throughout the body.

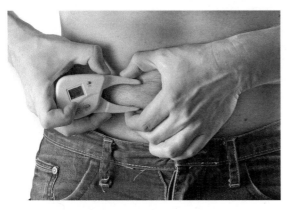

◀ FIGURE 1.2
Man measuring body fat with calipers.

SOURCE: Photograph by Ivica Drusany.

There are number of skinfold-measurement equations, each of which is tailored to the characteristics of different groups (old vs. young, athletes vs. nonathletes, etc.). The need to select the right equation for your characteristics, consistency in how measurements are taken, and experience level in using the calipers all contribute to variability in results. As a result, you may find that looking at how your measurements change over time to be most useful.

Hydrostatic weighing compares an individual's weight on land versus that under water and is thought by many to be the most accurate method for evaluating body composition. It requires specialized equipment and someone with expertise to perform the test, however, and is costly. Moreover, some would consider the process to be somewhat uncomfortable.

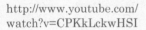
A new obesity measurement system, the **body volume index** (BVI), was devised in 2000 and uses body-scanning technology to measure BMI, waist circumference, and waist-to-hip ratio. It analyzes both body composition and how fat is distributed. It also takes ethnicity, gender, and age into consideration. The Body Benchmark Study, a collaborative international research project, was conducted between 2007 and 2010 to assess BVI and the scanning technology it uses. It's too early to tell whether or when it will replace BMI as a screening tool for obesity, but experts are excited by its potential.

5. What is the normal percentage of body fat for adults?

The normal percentage of body fat varies by gender and age, but experts don't necessarily agree on recommended ranges. Table 1.2 provides one set of guidelines for normal adult body-fat ranges.

TABLE 1.2 Healthy adult body-fat ranges

ADULT BODY-FAT RANGES		
	< Age 30	Age 30 and above
Males	14–20 percent	17–23 percent
Females	17–24 percent	20–27 percent

SOURCE: Girish Gadkari, *A Win over Obesity* (Navi Mumbai, India: Shroff Publishers & Distributors, 2005), 5.

In general, women can tolerate body fat better than men. In females, excess body fat is distributed as subcutaneous fat in the thighs, buttocks, and breasts—that is, gynoid obesity, or a pear-shaped body. (Following menopause, however, many women tend to undergo a redistribution of their body fat to the abdominal region.) In males, excess fat is stored in the abdominal cavity and as abdominal subcutaneous fat (android obesity, or an apple-shaped body). Android obesity is associated with an increased risk for obesity-related illnesses like heart disease and diabetes. Figure 1.3 illustrates the difference in body-fat distribution in the two body types.

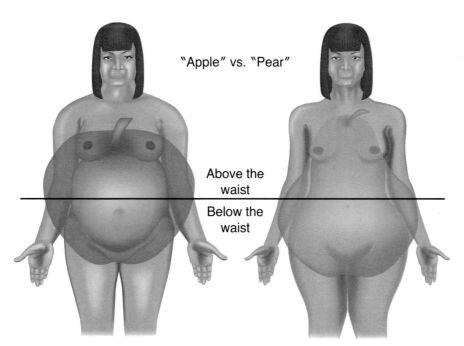

"Apple" vs. "Pear"

Above the waist

Below the waist

▲ FIGURE 1.3
Apple and pear body shapes.

6. What is the main cause of obesity?

People gain weight when their calorie intake exceeds the energy requirements of their bodies for physical activity and for growth. Globally, diets now include more energy-dense foods that are high in sugar, fat, and salt. At the same time, physical activity has decreased. The body accumulates these extra calories in the form of fat tissue, and if the imbalance between calorie intake and energy use continues, an individual can become obese over time.

A nutritional, or food, **calorie** is the amount of heat or energy required to raise the temperature of one kilogram of water by one degree Celsius. In nutrition, the term *calorie* refers to a **large calorie** (abbreviated **Cal**), as opposed to the **small calorie** (abbreviated **cal**) referenced in other scientific contexts. Nutritionists use *calorie* interchangeably with the term **kilocalorie** (abbreviated **kcal**).

DEFINITION

Calories give us energy to carry out different body functions. The metabolizable energy per gram of protein is 4 kcal, fat is 9 kcal, carbohydrate is 4 kcal, and alcohol is 7 kcal.

Small overages can add up to significant surpluses: 100 extra calories each day translates into 36,500 extra calories in a year. An excess of 7500 calories over time can form more than two pounds of fat, which will be deposited in the body if not used.

7. What other factors contribute to obesity?

Genetic factors, socioeconomic status, environment, access to health education, lack of sleep, stress, diet, and activity level can all play a role in the development of obesity. Food habits in a family matter a lot in the development of obesity in family members.

Other contributing factors include hormonal imbalance (for example, hypothyroidism), some medication like steroids, oral contraceptives, anxiolytic drugs (drugs used for reducing anxiety and tension), and some longstanding illnesses or treatment plans that require bed rest.

Childbearing can cause weight gain and may result in obesity in the long term if excess weight is not lost between successive pregnancies. Perimenopausal women also are likely to gain weight gradually, and if the weight gain is not addressed during this period, they are likely to be candidates for developing obesity as menopause sets in. A modified lifestyle, which includes diet restriction, exercise, and stress management, is the only solution. There is a tendency to attribute large gains in weight to menopause, but a gain of more than 8–13 pounds in the five years after menopause is likely due to a sedentary lifestyle and excess calories.

Although obesity is quite common in the middle-aged population (i.e., those 30–50 years old), it is also found increasingly in children (even infants) and adolescents. When one parent is obese, the chance that the child will become obese is 40 percent. When both parents are obese, the incidence can be as high as 80 percent.

Researchers currently are exploring whether other factors (food additives, processed food, how the body processes fructose versus glucose, etc.) may be at least partly responsible for the increase in obesity worldwide.

 ON THE WEB

For more information on rates of obesity in the United States, visit:

http://www.cdc.gov/obesity/data/adult.html

8. How prevalent is obesity?

According to the latest data available from the Centers for Disease Control and Prevention (CDC), more than 35 percent of adults and almost 17 percent of children and adolescents in the United States were obese in 2009–2010, although the incidence of obesity varies substantially among racial and socioeconomic groups.[2] According to the WHO, worldwide obesity has more than doubled since 1980.[3]

For an interactive map of obesity rates around the globe, visit:

http://gamapserver.who.int/gho/interactive_charts/ncd/risk_factors/overweight_obesity/atlas.html

For a closer look at the causes of the obesity epidemic and some of its consequences, visit:

http://www.uctv.tv/shows/The-Skinny-on-Obesity-Ep-1-An-Epidemic-for-Every-Body-23305

Obesity in Children and Adolescents

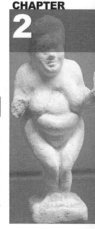

CHAPTER 2

9. How can I tell if my child's obese?

Body composition changes as children grow and is different for boys and girls, so **growth charts** are used in conjunction with BMI to determine whether a child is overweight or obese.[4] Growth charts classify children of the same age and gender into groups, or **percentiles**, which show how children compare to their peers in terms of weight and height (see Figure 2.1).

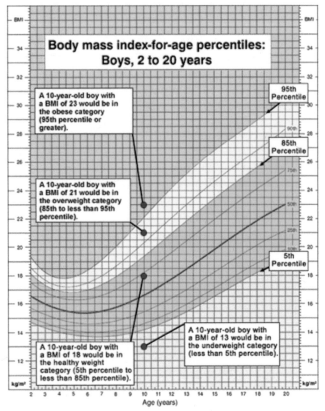

Body mass index-for-age percentiles:
Boys, 2 to 20 years

95th Percentile

A 10-year-old boy with a BMI of 23 would be in the obese category (95th percentile or greater).

85th Percentile

A 10-year-old boy with a BMI of 21 would be in the overweight category (85th to less than 95th percentile).

5th Percentile

A 10-year-old boy with a BMI of 13 would be in the underweight category (less than 5th percentile).

A 10-year-old boy with a BMI of 18 would be in the healthy weight category (5th percentile to less than 85th percentile).

Age (years)

SOURCE: Centers for Disease Control and Prevention, BMI-for-Age Growth Chart, http://www.cdc.gov/healthyweight/assessing/bmi/childrens_bmi/about_childrens_bmi.html

To see CDC growth charts, visit:

http://www.cdc.gov/growthcharts/clinical_charts.htm#Set1

ON THE WEB

To see WHO growth charts, visit:

http://www.cdc.gov/growthcharts/who_charts.htm

For guidelines on using growth charts, visit:

http://pediatrics.about.com/cs/growthcharts2/l/aa050802a.htm

Grouping children into percentiles makes it easier to see where an individual child falls on the chart and to follow whether that position remains consistent through time. As the child grows, drastic changes in position—for example, a child who has been in the 50th percentile suddenly appearing in the 75th percentile—may be a cause for concern.

The CDC recommends that clinicians use CDC growth charts for children and adolescents ages 2–19, and World

Health Organization (WHO) growth charts for children under 24 months.[5] Those with a BMI at or above the 85th percentile and lower than the 95th percentile are classified as overweight, while those with a BMI at or above the 95th percentile are considered obese.

For the CDC BMI calculator (ages 2–19), visit:

http://apps.nccd.cdc.gov/dnpabmi/

10. How prevalent is childhood obesity?

According to the CDC, "obesity now affects 17 percent of all children and adolescents [ages 2–19] in the United States—triple the rate from just one generation ago."[6] However, obesity rates show significant variation among racial and income groups and by state: Hispanic boys, non-Hispanic black girls, and low-income children are all disproportionately affected.

For more information on how obesity rates vary by demographic group and geographic location, visit:

http://www.cdc.gov/obesity/data/childhood.html

For highlights of a Wayne University study on obesity in children younger than 24 months, visit:

http://research.wayne.edu/rwnews/article.php?id=791

11. What factors contribute to childhood obesity?

As with adults, an imbalance between calorie intake and the body's energy requirements for physical activity and for growth can lead to obesity, but other factors have an impact as well.

Family history and lifestyle

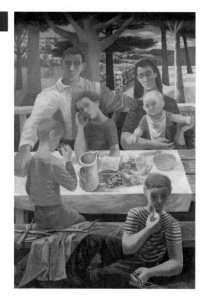

As noted in Question 7, when one parent is obese, the chance that the child will become obese is 40 percent. When both the parents are obese, the incidence can be as high as 80 percent. Genes, however, only determine the number of fat cells and the distribution of fat in tissues. The family's attitude towards food, its social and economic status, and how the children in the family are educated about health are more important than genetic factors in determining whether a child will become obese.

Social pressures, depression, frustration, boredom, lack of affection, family troubles, etc., can lead adults to treat food as a drug, and children may follow the example of family members and acquire the same habits. Parents also can fall into the trap of letting children eat sweets and other junk food to gain their affection, and the time pressures faced by parents when both are working can result in a tendency to rely on fast food. In addition, many parents don't believe that a child being overweight is a medical problem, and may view even a normal diet as a starvation regime. In short, psychological and psychosocial factors within the family are very significant in the onset of childhood obesity.

Nutrition during pregnancy

For results of a recent University of South Australia study on how nutrition in pregnancy affects a child's weight in later life, visit:

http://w3.unisa.edu.au/news/2006/201106.asp

For more on how a mother's nutrition affects her child's chances for becoming obese, visit:

http://www.uctv.tv/shows/The-Skinny-on-Obesity-Ep-5-Generation-XL-23719

For additional pregnancy weight-gain guidelines and nutrition tips, see Document 2.1.PregWeight.

During the last three months of pregnancy, the human fetus adds 14–16 percent of the fat in the body, and the fat cells produced during this period last for life. It's important to pay attention to the effect nutrition during pregnancy has on the number and size of the fat cells in the fetus. Eating too much during pregnancy is more likely to produce infants with higher birth weights and larger fat cells (and possibly an increased number of fat cells). These babies tend to become obese children, which in turn may predispose them to obesity in adulthood.

As mentioned in Question 7, gaining too much weight during pregnancy also affects a mother's chances of becoming obese over time, particularly if excess weight is not lost after childbirth. Total weight gain recommended by the National Academy of Sciences' Institute of Medicine varies according to the mother's BMI and whether she is carrying twins, but a woman of normal weight who is not carrying twins should limit weight gain to 25–35 pounds.

Bottle feeding vs. breastfeeding

A number of studies have shown an association between breastfeeding and a reduced risk of obesity for children, but research has yet to establish a causal relationship. (In part, this is because conducting the necessary randomized clinical trials would be unethical, because infants placed in non-breastfeeding groups would be deprived of the established health benefits of breastfeeding.) Several biological reasons could be responsible for such a relationship, however:

* Breastfed infants rely on internal signals from their bodies to tell them they're full and that it's time to stop eating. They may be able to control their consumption more effectively, therefore, than formula-fed infants, who may instead be relying on the person feeding them to tell them when the feeding is over.

* Formula-fed babies have a higher concentration of insulin in their blood and experience a longer insulin response time than those that are breastfed. Experts have established that higher concentrations of insulin cue the body to increase fat deposits, increasing weight gain.

* Concentrations of leptin (a hormone that is key to regulating appetite and metabolism) may be affected by breastfeeding.

For more information on breastfeeding and obesity, see Document 2.2. BreastFeed.

According to research published in the *International Journal of Obesity*, breastfeeding may also have an impact on the mother's chances of becoming obese: the study showed that on average, BMI was 1 percent lower for every six months of breastfeeding.[7]

Early nutrition

It's normal for children to add fat cells in first few years of life and between ages 9 and 13, but the number multiplies rapidly when a child starts gaining weight at early age. If the child is obese, these cells will be larger, as they are for all obese persons. Once fat cells are formed the child has them for life.

For a guide to infant nutrition, see Document 2.3.InfantNutr.

There are two types of obesity: hyperplastic (an increased number of fat cells, which can be of normal or increased size) and hypertrophic (a normal number of fat cells of increased size). Hyperplastic obesity is more likely when the onset of obesity occurs in childhood. When carried to adulthood, hyperplastic obesity is harder to manage for the physician and the patient because it becomes difficult for the patient to maintain weight loss. (Although hyperplastic obesity is quite common in people who have been obese since early childhood, it can still occur later in life.)

Overfeeding in the first year of life increases the number of fat cells. Researchers now also think that introducing solid food to formula-fed newborns under four months old can lead to obesity by age three (the same did not appear to be true for breast-fed infants).[8] Breastfeeding for a reasonable length of time and postponing the introduction of solid food seem to reduce the risk of development of obesity in young children.[9]

For an early-nutrition family checklist, visit:

http://nrckids.org/
nutritionchecklist.pdf

ON THE WEB

Childhood eating patterns

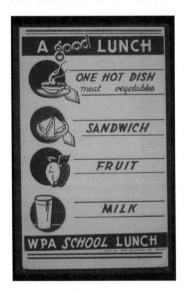

As noted in the previous section, hyperplastic obesity (the kind that usually starts in childhood) is characterized by an increased number of fat cells in fat tissue depots. When people with hyperplastic obesity lose weight, the size of the cells decreases but the number remains constant. It may be useful to think of fat cells like hungry animals: when deprived of food they shrink in size, but the moment food is made available to them they attack it with double the force and store fat in themselves at a faster speed. Individuals with hyperplastic obesity must expend a lot of effort to lose weight, and even more to keep it off, because they carry more fat cells than a person of normal weight and that number will always remain the same. Reducing the size of fat cells only gives temporary results, which is why these individuals end up dieting constantly to maintain their weight.

For a look at how preschoolers learning about healthy lifestyles can help the whole family, see Video 2.1.Preschool.

ON THE DVD

Weight reduction programs should start early, therefore, before children reach a degree of obesity that is characterized by an increase in the number of fat cells. If eating and physical activity patterns are to be changed (and can be changed), early intervention will prove more beneficial.

Parents who are obese themselves should think seriously about the problem of obesity in their children and act accordingly, because between 50 and 85 percent of obese adolescents become obese adults. For children who are obese at age 12, the odds are 4:1 against attaining ideal body weight (IBW); for those who are obese after adolescence, the odds are 28:1 against attaining IBW.[10]

Endocrinal Abnormality

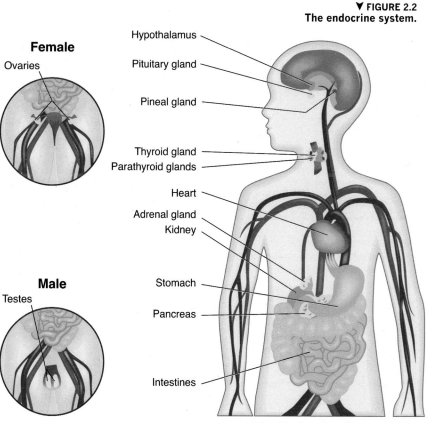

▼ FIGURE 2.2
The endocrine system.

Female
Ovaries

Male
Testes

Hypothalamus
Pituitary gland
Pineal gland
Thyroid gland
Parathyroid glands
Heart
Adrenal gland
Kidney
Stomach
Pancreas
Intestines

The Endocrine System

In a small percentage of the population, childhood obesity can be caused by factors other than a positive energy balance. If there is no family history of obesity and the development of obesity coincides with a cessation of growth in height, further diagnostic studies will be needed to rule out endocrinal dysfunctions (see Figure 2.2). A child of average or above average height who carries excess weight is invariably a case of nonglandular obesity.

Society and Environment

The lifestyle changes that have taken place in the United States (and elsewhere in the world) over the last few decades have had an impact on children as well as adults. Many children now prefer to watch TV or play on the computer during leisure time instead of playing outdoor games with friends. Community safety concerns and lack of access to physical activity programs at day care centers and schools also affect how active children are.

For an overview of major causes of childhood obesity, see Document 2.4.GrowProb.

ON THE DVD

For a look at how the Western diet has increased the incidence of obesity in children, see:

ON THE WEB

http://www.ucsf.edu/news/2006/08/5459/childhood-obesity-caused-toxic-environment-western-diets-study-says

Meanwhile, the decrease in physical activity has been accompanied by an increase in portion sizes and in the availability of high calorie foods and sugar drinks, all of which have contributed to the rise in childhood obesity.

12. What physical effects does being overweight have on a child?

According to the CDC, in the near term "obese youth are more likely to have risk factors for cardiovascular disease, such as high cholesterol or high blood pressure . . . [and are] more likely to have prediabetes, a condition in which blood glucose levels indicate a high risk for development of diabetes." In the longer term, "[c]hildren and adolescents who are obese are likely to be obese as adults and are therefore more at risk for adult health problems such as heart disease, type 2 diabetes, stroke, several types of cancer, and osteoarthritis. One study showed that children who became obese as early as age two were more likely to be obese as adults . . . Children and adolescents who are obese are [also] at greater risk for bone and joint problems, sleep apnea, and social and psychological problems such as stigmatization and poor self-esteem."[11] Figure 2.3 provides a visual summary of the complications—both physiological and psychological—of childhood obesity.

The immediate risk factor in an obese child is mechanical in nature. Deformation of the spine or the long bones of the limbs (such as knock-knees or flat feet) are quite marked in obese children, and these deformities are more common if the obesity is accompanied by vitamin

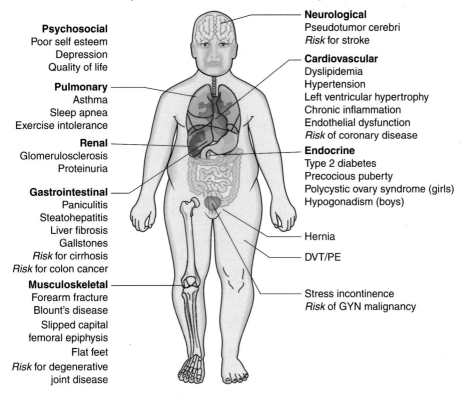

Complications of Childhood Obesity

Psychosocial
Poor self esteem
Depression
Quality of life

Pulmonary
Asthma
Sleep apnea
Exercise intolerance

Renal
Glomerulosclerosis
Proteinuria

Gastrointestinal
Paniculitis
Steatohepatitis
Liver fibrosis
Gallstones
Risk for cirrhosis
Risk for colon cancer

Musculoskeletal
Forearm fracture
Blount's disease
Slipped capital
femoral epiphysis
Flat feet
Risk for degenerative
joint disease

Neurological
Pseudotumor cerebri
Risk for stroke

Cardiovascular
Dyslipidemia
Hypertension
Left ventricular hypertrophy
Chronic inflammation
Endothelial dysfunction
Risk of coronary disease

Endocrine
Type 2 diabetes
Precocious puberty
Polycystic ovary syndrome (girls)
Hypogonadism (boys)

Hernia

DVT/PE

Stress incontinence
Risk of GYN malignancy

D or calcium deficiencies from diets rich in sucrose and fats and poor in proteins, trace elements, and vitamins.

Obese children also suffer from frequent attacks of tonsillitis and respiratory infections that take a longer time to respond to treatment than the same attacks in children of normal weight because of a low resistance to fighting infections. These children also get tired quickly even when engaged in normal activities and can't concentrate on schoolwork as well as children who are not overweight. Sleepiness, irritability, and mood changes are common among overweight children and they have a tendency to be more attention seeking as well. Obesity health risks for children and adults are discussed in detail in Chapter 3.

13. What psychological effects does being overweight have on a child?

Physical inactivity and a large body size have a negative psychological impact on overweight children, whose large size can give them a false sense of strength that's missing in their self-awareness. There's no doubt that obesity is not a pleasant experience for a child, and even less so for an adolescent. Overweight children often are teased (or bullied) by friends, relatives, and at school, which can lead to depression, anxiety, and low self-esteem. These children also can experience apathy and lack of self-confidence and can find it difficult to get attached to other people, leading to isolation and detachment from the immediate environment. Moreover, coping with being overweight may begin a vicious cycle in which children avoid physical activity or eat to manage their boredom or emotional issues, adding to their weight in the process. Obesity in childhood thus becomes an extremely complicated social, psychological, and physiological phenomenon.

CHAPTER 3

Obesity and Health

14. What are the health risks associated with obesity?

There are a number of medical complications associated with obesity, many of which can have a serious effect on quality of life and lifespan (see Figure 3.1). We describe some of the more common conditions in the sections that follow.

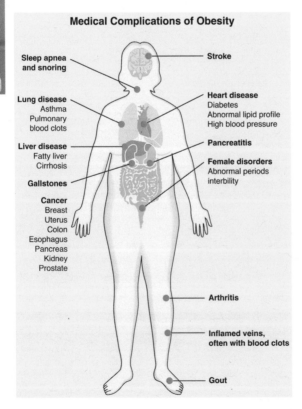

Medical Complications of Obesity

Sleep apnea and snoring

Stroke

Lung disease
Asthma
Pulmonary
blood clots

Heart disease
Diabetes
Abnormal lipid profile
High blood pressure

Liver disease
Fatty liver
Cirrhosis

Pancreatitis

Female disorders
Abnormal periods
interbility

Gallstones

Cancer
Breast
Uterus
Colon
Esophagus
Pancreas
Kidney
Prostate

Arthritis

Inflamed veins,
often with blood clots

Gout

◄ FIGURE 3.1
Health risks
associated with
obesity.

Obesity frequently is associated with an abnormal level of blood lipids. Blood lipids are mainly fatty acids, which provide fuel for the body, and cholesterol, which is necessary for a cell membrane's fluidity and permeability. Elevated levels of triglycerides—a blood lipid that stores unused calories—and cholesterol are quite common in obese individuals, as are lowered HDL (high-density lipoproteins, or good cholesterol) levels and increased LDL (low-density lipoproteins, or bad cholesterol) levels. A high fat diet, consumption of large quantities of alcohol and sweets, and lack of exercise are often behind abnormal cholesterol levels.

HDL is called *good cholesterol* because it carries excess cholesterol back to the liver where it's flushed from the body, helping to prevent clogged arteries. LDL is termed *bad cholesterol* because it tends to stick to blood vessel walls, contributing to blockages (see Figure 3.2).

Overweight individuals have a significantly increased rate of hyperlipidemia (high blood lipid levels, including cholesterol

▼ **FIGURE 3.2**
HDL vs. LDL cholesterol.

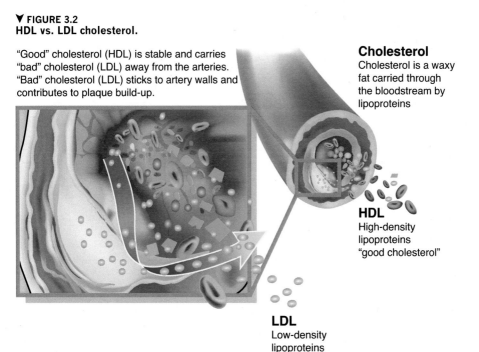

"Good" cholesterol (HDL) is stable and carries "bad" cholesterol (LDL) away from the arteries. "Bad" cholesterol (LDL) sticks to artery walls and contributes to plaque build-up.

Cholesterol
Cholesterol is a waxy fat carried through the bloodstream by lipoproteins

HDL
High-density lipoproteins "good cholesterol"

LDL
Low-density lipoproteins "bad cholesterol"

For more information about hyperlipidemia, visit:

http//www.vascularweb.org/vascularhealth/Pages/hyperlipidemia.aspx

 ON THE WEB

In the United States, lipids are measured in terms of milligrams per deciliter of blood (mg/dL). In Canada and in most of Europe, lipids are measured in terms of millimoles per liter of blood (mmol/L).

NOTE

and/or triglycerides) and **hypercholesterolemia** (high cholesterol levels) compared to individuals of normal weight.[12] Not all obese people have these conditions, however, while some individuals with normal weight and good eating habits do.

Blood tests can be used to generate **lipid profiles**, which show levels of HDL, LDL, total cholesterol, and triglycerides.

Medical professionals use lipid profiles to evaluate whether lipid levels pose a potential risk to cardiovascular health. Table 3.1 shows U.S. cardiovascular risk categories for different cholesterol and triglyceride levels.

TABLE 3.1 Evaluating cardiovascular risk: blood lipid levels

	LOWER RISK	BORDERLINE HIGH	HIGH RISK
Total Cholesterol	< 200	200–239	240+
HDL	> 60	40–59	Men < 40 Women < 50
LDL	< 130	130–159	160+
Triglycerides	< 150	150–199	200+

Source: Based on American Heart Association recommendations, "What Do My Cholesterol Levels Mean?", http://www.heart.org/idc/groups/heart-public/@wcm/@hcm/documents/downloadable/ucm_300301.pdf

Because HDL promotes cardiovascular health, the ratio of total cholesterol to HDL provides information about risks to cardiovascular health. This ratio is calculated by dividing your total cholesterol value by your HDL value. For example, a total cholesterol value of 220 would be considered a borderline high risk to cardiovascular health (see Table 3.1). When paired with a favorable HDL level of 65, however, the ratio of 220/65 (3.4) paints a more positive picture of heart health (see Table 3.2). However, the American Heart Association recommends that health care providers use the absolute numbers, as it considers them more useful in determining appropriate treatment courses.

TABLE 3.2 Evaluating cardiovascular risk: total cholesterol/HDL ratio

RISK	RATIO
Low	3.5 or lower
Average	3.6 < 5
High	5+

Source: Based on American Heart Association recommendations, http://www.
heart.org/HEARTORG/Conditions/Cholesterol/AboutCholesterol/What-Your-
Cholesterol-Levels-Mean_UCM_305562_Article.jsp

The body also produces its own cholesterol, which can contribute to the development of both hyperlipidemia and hypercholesterolemia. Genetic predisposition is a major factor in developing these conditions.

ON THE DVD

For information about lowering cholesterol with the Therapeutic Lifestyle Changes (TLC) program, see Document 3.1.CholTLC.

Hyperlipidemia is responsible for **atheromatous plaque deposits** (fatty deposits in arteries) on the inside linings of blood vessels, including coronary arteries and cerebral blood vessels. These deposits cause arteries that supply blood to the heart and brain to thicken, a condition known as **atherosclerosis** that can ultimately lead to a heart attack or stroke (see Figure 3.3).[13]

Coronary Heart Disease

Obese persons are more likely than lean or nonobese individuals to be the victims of **coronary heart disease** (CHD). It's interesting to note, however, that being underweight is equally likely to cause CHD.

CLOSER LOOK

For a comprehensive review of CHD that includes causes, symptoms, and available treatments, see *Heart Disease and Health* from Mercury Learning and Information:

CHD develops from atherosclerosis in the arteries of the heart (see previous section on abnormal lipid

http://www.merclearning.com/titles/Heart_Disease.html

levels). When plaque builds up inside the arteries that supply blood to the heart, it limits blood flow over time and can lead to heart attacks (see Figure 3.4).

Individuals in obesity class II who are 35–45 years old have double the risk of nonobese persons in the same age group of death from coronary heart disease. For class II individuals 50–60 years old there is a threefold increase in the chances of dying from CHD.

TOOLS

For a 10-year CHD risk calculator, visit:

http://www.mcw.edu/calculators/Coronary-Heart-Disease-Risk.htm#.UE8YO44TufQ

▼ FIGURE 3.3
Atherosclerosis.
(A) A normal artery with normal blood flow. (B) An artery with plaque buildup.

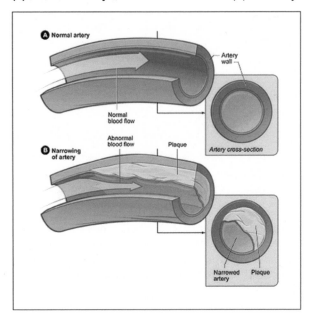

SOURCE: National Heart, Lung, and Blood Institute, National Institutes of Health, U.S. Department of Health and Human Services, http://www.nhlbi.nih.gov/health/health-topics/topics/atherosclerosis/

▼ FIGURE 3.4
Heart with muscle damage and a blocked artery.
(A) Dead heart muscle from heart attack. (B) Blocked coronary artery.

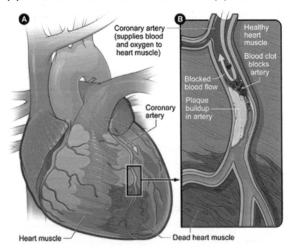

SOURCE: National Heart, Lung, and Blood Institute, National Institutes of Health, U.S. Department of Health and Human Services, http://www.nhlbi.nih.gov/health/health-topics/topics/heartattack/

High blood pressure and **hypertension** are both associated with being overweight, and the increasing prevalence of obesity has been accompanied by an increased prevalence

According to the CDC, high blood pressure contributes to nearly 1000 deaths a day.

of hypertension. Technically high blood pressure is a symptom, while hypertension is the condition of chronic elevated blood pressure, but the terms are used almost interchangeably.

Blood pressure (BP for short) is expressed in terms of systolic pressure (the pressure when your heart beats) over diastolic pressure (the pressure when your heart rests between beats), and is considered normal when it's less than 120/80 as measured in millimeters of mercury hemoglobin (mmHg), the units used to measure BP (see Table 3.3).

TABLE 3.3 Blood pressure levels

BLOOD PRESSURE LEVELS		
	Systolic Level	Diastolic Level
Normal	90–119	60–79
Prehypertension	120–139	80–89
High	140+	90+

SOURCE: Based on American Heart Association blood pressure categories, http://www.heart.org/HEARTORG/Conditions/HighBloodPressure/About HighBloodPressure/Understanding-Blood-Pressure-Readings_UCM_301764_ Article.jsp

Obese individuals with normal blood pressure are more likely to develop high BP than individuals with normal BP who fall in a normal weight range. Weight reduction has a remarkable influence on lowering elevated BP. A weight reduction of about 20–30 pounds can reduce systolic blood pressure by 20–25 mmHg and diastolic blood pressure by 10–15 mmHg.

If there are no immediate dangers to the health of a person with high BP, weight reduction should be tried before starting any medication. For individuals on medication to control BP, weight reduction allows physicians either to reduce the dose or to stop the medicine altogether once the weight is reduced. Both

For additional information and resources about high blood pressure and hypertension, see Document 3.2.HighBP.

For a pocket guide to high blood pressure in children, see Document 3.3.HighBPChild.

overweight and normal weight people are likely to develop hypertension if there is a family history of high blood pressure.

Diabetes

Diabetes is a disease characterized by too much glucose (sugar) in the blood. Glucose is the main source of energy for cells and is manufactured by the liver and the muscles, and metabolized by the body from the food we eat. The pancreas makes the hormone insulin to help glucose get into your cells and to keep blood sugar levels from getting too high. If insulin levels are too low, blood sugar levels will be too high.

There are three main kinds of diabetes:

Type 1 diabetes (previously known as **juvenile diabetes** and also known as **insulin-dependent diabetes**) means the pancreas can't make insulin because of a problem caused by the body's immune system. Type 1 diabetes usually (but not always) develops during childhood and young adulthood.

Gestational diabetes sometimes occurs during the later stages of pregnancy because of hormones or a shortage of insulin. It's usually temporary, although women who've had it have a greater chance of developing type 2 diabetes later on. Woman who are overweight have an increased risk of developing gestational diabetes.

Type 2 diabetes (also known as **non-insulin dependent diabetes**, or **NIDD**) is the most common form of the disease in the United States. According to the NIH it accounts for 90–95 percent of people diagnosed with diabetes, 80 percent of whom are overweight or obese.[14] Type 2 diabetes is also more prevalent in some racial groups than others. Incidence of type 2 diabetes is increasing rapidly worldwide due to changes in nutrition and lifestyle.

For an overview of diabetes, see Document 3.4.DiabOver.

For a diabetes fact sheet, see Document 3.5.DiabFacts.

ON THE DVD

Type 2 diabetes usually starts with insulin resistance, in which cells lose their ability to use insulin to absorb glucose, fatty acids, and amino acids. As a result, blood glucose levels rise. The pancreas initially tries to compensate by making more insulin but eventually is unable to secrete enough for the body's needs. Obesity plays an important role in the onset of type 2 diabetes in people who are genetically predisposed to this disease. Studies of identical twins have shown that if one twin develops type 2 diabetes, the other almost always develops it as well, irrespective of weight.

Experts aren't certain whether obesity alone can cause type 2 diabetes in a person who has no family history of the disease. Weight reduction obviously will have a very positive effect on individuals with the disease,

To learn about diabetes prevention, see Video 3.1.Diabetes.

and weight reduction and lifestyle changes definitely will help those with a family history of type 2 diabetes reduce the chances of developing it. Obese individuals with a family history of diabetes need to take the need to reduce their weight very seriously. According to the CDC, diabetes is the seventh leading cause of death in the United States, a major cause of heart disease and stroke, and the leading cause of kidney failure, nontraumatic lower-limb amputation, and new cases of blindness among adults.[15]

Osteoarthritis

▼ FIGURE 3.5
Osteoarthritis of knee joint.

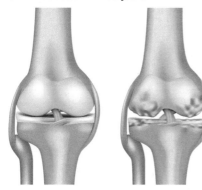

Healthy knee joint   Osteoarthritis

SOURCE: Diagram by Alila Sao Mai.

Osteoarthritis (also known as degenerative arthritis) is a condition caused by degeneration of the cartilage and bone of joints. When the cartilage cushioning joints wears away, bones rub together, resulting in pain, swelling, and stiffness in the affected joints (see Figure 3.5). Many people develop osteoarthritis in middle age simply through wear and tear on the joints, and by age 70 most people have some symptoms.

Obese individuals (particularly women) are prone to developing osteoarthritis in their weight-bearing joints, such as hips, knees, ankles, and feet—and even in their hands— later in life. Weight reduction will

Osteoarthritis is different from rheumatoid arthritis, an autoimmune disease in which the body's immune system attacks soft tissue and joints, causing inflammation of the joints and surrounding tissue.

not reverse any damage done, but it will definitely relieve the pain associated with the disease and increase mobility. Weight reduction prior to hip or knee replacement surgery is essential for a successful outcome, and, needless to say, maintaining an ideal weight after surgery is equally important in achieving benefit from replacement surgeries.

For results of an August 2009 Boston University study that links being overweight with an increased risk of osteoarthritis, visit:

http://www.youtube.com/watch?v=FyAFsR-uxy8

For more information about PCOS and its associated conditions, visit:

http://www.youtube.com/watch?v=-DMflo_ogho

Obesity has adverse effects on reproductive functions. Women who are extremely underweight or overweight are likely to show some irregularities in menstrual cycle and can even fail to ovulate normally. **Polycystic ovary syndrome (PCOS)**, a condition in which a woman's periods are indefinitely delayed or absent, is many times associated with obesity. Women with PCOS are predisposed to elevated cholesterol and triglyceride levels, have an increased risk of developing type 2 diabetes and endometrial cancer, and may also have problems with fertility. Substantial weight reduction can improve ovarian function dramatically in women with irregular cycles.

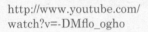
Problems during pregnancy and labor

Morbidly obese females who become pregnant can develop complications like bleeding, **preeclampsia** (a condition that results in elevated BP, also known as toxemia), and gestational diabetes (see the previous section on diabetes). Normal labor also sometimes becomes difficult for an obese woman, requiring that a caesarian section be performed.

For more on how obesity complicates pregnancy and labor, visit:

http://www.youtube.com/watch?v=NBpwHwYb8Kw

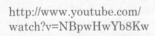
Obstructive sleep apnea

The word *apnea* means "without breath" in Greek.

People with **obstructive sleep apnea (OSA)** experience successive pauses in breath while sleeping due to a blockage in the upper respiratory tract.

This airway obstruction is caused by soft tissue in the airway collapsing, which itself can be caused by reduced muscle tone (see Figure 3.6).

The typical person with OSA is overweight. Over time OSA can cause a number of problems for people suffering from it, including daytime

▼ FIGURE 3.6
Obstructive sleep apnea.

Normal Breathing

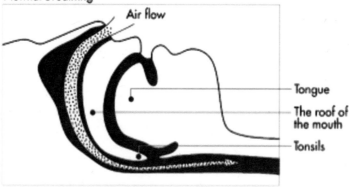

Sleep Apnea

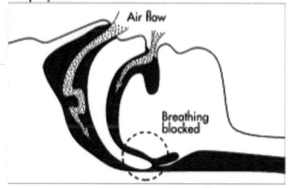

SOURCE: National Institute of Neurological Disorders and Stroke, National Institutes of Health, U.S. Dept. of Health and Human Services, http://www.ninds.nih.gov/education/brochures/Brain-Basics-Sleep-6-10-08-pdf-508.pdf, 11.

sleepiness, irritability, depression, as well as an increased risk for hypertension, CHD, and stroke. Research suggests that losing weight can significantly improve sleep apnea.

For results of a study showing how weight loss improves OSA, visit:

http://www.webmd.com/sleep-disorders/sleep-apnea/news/20090928/weight loss-helps-sleep-apnea

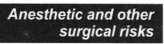

Anesthetic and other surgical risks

Both surgeons and anesthesiologists face challenges when treating obese patients. Obesity interferes with a smooth anesthetic procedure during surgery by complicating even simple monitoring tasks that are essential for preserving the health and well-being of all patients. It may be difficult, for example, to find blood pressure cuffs to fit obese

For more information on how obesity complicates the administration of anesthesia during surgery, visit:

ON THE WEB

http://www.youtube.com/watch?v=jieCaX6LIU0

For some postoperative complications faced by the morbidly obese, visit:

http://www.livestrong.com/article/29724-morbid-obesity-surgical-complications/

patients, and locating veins can be harder as well. Anesthesiologists also will almost certainly find it harder to determine appropriate doses of drugs and may be limited in the drugs they can use. The higher incidence of obstructive sleep apnea in obese individuals (see the previous section on OSA) makes the management of airways harder and makes reduced airflow and oxygen in sedated patients more likely.

Obese patients present similar challenges to their surgeons during surgery and are at a significantly higher risk for postoperative complications, such as blood clots in the lungs, heart attacks, wound infection, and nerve injury.

Increased cancer risk

Being overweight is associated with an increased risk of certain kinds of cancer, including postmenopausal breast and uterine cancer in women, colorectal cancer in men, and kidney and esophageal cancer in both sexes (see Figure 3.7).

▼ FIGURE 3.7
Obesity-linked cancers.

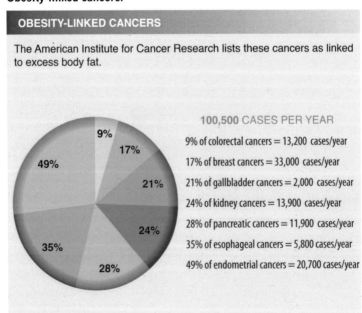

OBESITY-LINKED CANCERS

The American Institute for Cancer Research lists these cancers as linked to excess body fat.

100,500 CASES PER YEAR

9% of colorectal cancers = 13,200 cases/year

17% of breast cancers = 33,000 cases/year

21% of gallbladder cancers = 2,000 cases/year

24% of kidney cancers = 13,900 cases/year

28% of pancreatic cancers = 11,900 cases/year

35% of esophageal cancers = 5,800 cases/year

49% of endometrial cancers = 20,700 cases/year

Obese individuals appear to have about twice the risk of developing these cancers as overweight individuals. Meanwhile, one study estimates that if existing obesity trends continue, the result could be about 500,000 additional cases of cancer in the United States by 2030.[16]

For information on cancer risk associated with excess weight, visit:

http://www.youtube.com/watch?v=w8ZW9YdHgFM

For more information on obesity and cancer risk, see Document 3.6.CancerFacts.

15. What challenges do obese people face with respect to exercise?

Obese individuals have obvious impediments to exercising, which is essential to good health and maintaining a healthy weight. Even normal-weight individuals can become tired or breathless when carrying a bag full of groceries or a heavy suitcase for a short distance or up a flight of stairs, and people who are obese carry a similar amount of extra weight with them wherever they go, making day-to-day activities difficult to manage.

Exercise can be an unpleasant experience for the obese for a number of reasons, including discomfort when walking due to joint problems, an inability to fit into equipment at the gym, and abuse from other people. Naturally enough, there can be a tendency to drop out from exercise programs, which of course contributes to accumulating extra weight.

Ways to overcome barriers to exercise are discussed in Chapter 7.

16. What are the psychological and social effects of obesity?

Obesity can be a serious handicap in the social, emotional, and professional life of an individual. Society tends to view people who are obese as weak-willed and lacking in self-discipline, and therefore unworthy of respect or consideration. Obese individuals are subject to weight-related lectures, disapproval, and abuse from friends, family, and strangers. Their size can interfere with routine activities—such as taking public transportation, getting on an airplane, or going to the movies—because the seats or other accommodations are too small. As a result of these difficulties and the negative attitudes toward them, many choose to limit their time in public. Taken together with the discrimination they face when applying for jobs and promotions, these factors can lead to anxiety, depression, and low self-esteem over time.

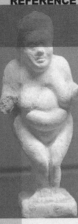

Part One Unlabeled Figures

Part One large opening figure and opening figure for chapters. Photograph of theater fat woman (2005) courtesy of Marie-Lan Nguyen, available online at http://commons.wikimedia.org/wiki/ File:Theater_fat_woman_Louvre_BC968bis.jpg

Part One small opening figure (page 3) and Question 4. Undated photograph of man measuring body fat with calipers by Ivica Drusany, available online at http://www.shutterstock.com/cat.mhtm l?searchterm=calipers+body+fat&search_group=&lang=en&search_ source=search_form%20-%20id=71313037&src=d9d61d34f898eabcb dae607e7bed76f9-1-1#id=71313037&src=1ca42dfe26af38cf0a754614 c960c4c1-1-1

Question 2. Photograph of U.S. President William Howard Taft by unidentified photographer (ca. 1908), Library of Congress, available online at http://www.loc.gov/pictures/item/96521946/

Question 3. Toyokuni Utagawa, *Higashi no kata Ichiriki* [The wrestler Ichiriki of the East Side] (ca. 1847), Library of Congress, available online at http://www.loc.gov/pictures/ item/2009615267/

Question 11 (Family history and lifestyle). Carol M. Highsmith, photograph of WPA mural, Cohen Building, Washington, D.C. (2008), Library of Congress, available online at http://www.loc.gov/pictures/ item/2010720417/

Question 11 (Bottle feeding vs. breastfeeding). Erik Hans Krause, "Nurse the Baby" WPA poster (between 1936 and 1938), Library of Congress, available online at http://www.loc.gov/pictures/ item/98516179/

Question 11 (Childhood eating patterns). Works Progress Administration (WPA) Oklahoma Art Project, school lunch poster (between 1936 and 1941), Library of Congress, available online at http://www.loc.gov/pictures/item/98517081/

Part One Additional Source Information

Figure 1.2. Undated photograph by Ivica Drusany, available online at http://www.shutterstock.com/cat.mhtml?searchterm=calipers+body+f at&search_group=&lang=en&search_source=search_form#id=713130 37&src=d9d61d34f898eabcbdae607e7bed76f9-1-1

Figure 3.5. Undated diagram by Alila Sao Mai, available online at http://www.shutterstock.com/cat.mhtml?lang=en&search_ source=search_form&version=llv1&anyorall=all&safesearch=1

&searchterm=Osteoarthritis&search_group=&orient=&search_
cat=&searchtermx=&photographer_name=&people_gender=&people_
age=&people_ethnicity=&people_number=&commercial_
ok=&color=&show_color_wheel=1#id=94626562

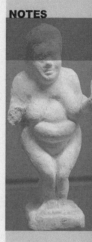

	Part One Notes

	Chapter 1

1. Centers for Disease Control and Prevention (CDC), "FastStats/
   Obesity and Overweight" (data as of 2009–2010), available online at
   http://www.cdc.gov/nchs/fastats/overwt.htm, August 23, 2012.

2. CDC, "Adult Obesity Facts," available online at http://www.cdc.gov/
   obesity/data/adult.html, August 23, 2012.

3. World Health Organization (WHO), *Obesity and Overweight* (Fact
   Sheet No. 311), available online at http://www.who.int/mediacentre/
   factsheets/fs311/en/, August 23, 2012.

	Chapter 2

4. BMI for children and adolescents is calculated as a weight-to-
   height ratio, just as it is for adults. For children under two years of
   age—who typically cannot stand well enough to measure height—a
   weight-to-length ratio is calculated.

5. For a detailed explanation of the CDC's rationale and the difference
   between WHO and CDC growth charts, see "Use of World Health
   Organization and CDC Growth Charts for Children Aged 0–59
   Months in the United States," available online at http://www.cdc.
   gov/mmwr/preview/mmwrhtml/rr5909a1.htm, August 28, 2012.

6. CDC, "Childhood Overweight and Obesity," available online at
   http://www.cdc.gov/obesity/childhood/index.html, August 28, 2012.

7. K. L. Bobrow et al., "Persistent Effects of Women's Parity and
   Breastfeeding Patterns on Their Body Mass Index: Results from
   the Million Women Study," *International Journal of Obesity*
   (advance online publication July 10, 2012), 1–6, available online at
   http://www.nature.com/ijo/journal/vaop/ncurrent/abs/ijo201276a.
   html, August 28, 2012. For a discussion of the study's results,
   see Kathleen Doheny, "Childbearing Is Linked to Larger Size,
   but Nursing Cuts the Odds, Study Finds," HealthDay (July 10,
   2012), available online at http://consumer.healthday.com/Article.
   asp?AID=666532, January 20, 2013.

8. Susanna Y. Huh et al., "Timing of Solid Food Introduction and Risk of Obesity in Preschool-Aged Children," *Pediatrics* 127:3 (2011), e544–e551, available online at http://pediatrics.aappublications.org/content/early/2011/02/07/peds.2010-0740.full.pdf+html, August 28, 2012. For a discussion of the study's results, see Crystal Phend, "Bottle-Fed Babies at Risk for Early Obesity," MedPage Today (February 7, 2011), available online at http://www.medpagetoday.com/Pediatrics/GeneralPediatrics/24723, August 28, 2012.

9. The American Academy of Pediatrics (AAP) recommends breastfeeding unless specifically contraindicated, and states further that "[p]ediatricians and parents should be aware that exclusive breastfeeding is sufficient to support optimal growth and development for approximately the first six months of life and provides continuing protection against diarrhea and respiratory tract infection. Breastfeeding should be continued for at least the first year of life and beyond for as long as mutually desired by mother and child." See AAP, "Breastfeeding and the Use of Human Milk," *Pediatrics* 115:2 (2005), 496–506, available online at http://pediatrics.aappublications.org/content/115/2/496.full.html#sec-12, August 28, 2012.

10. Lawrence S. Neinstein et al. (eds.), *Adolescent Health Care: A Practical Guide*, 5th ed. (Philadelphia, PA: Lippincott, Williams, and Wilkins, 2007), 470.

11. CDC, "Childhood Obesity Facts: Health Effects of Childhood Obesity," available online at http://www.cdc.gov/healthyyouth/obesity/facts.htm, August 30, 2012.

Chapter 3

12. Hypercholesterolemia and hyperlipidemia are terms that have been used interchangeably, but hyperlipidemia refers to high levels of any lipids in the bloodstream (including cholesterol and triglycerides), while hypercholesterolemia is a form of hyperlipidemia and refers only to high cholesterol levels in the blood.

13. Atherosclerosis is one of three types of arteriosclerosis, a general term for hardening of the arteries. In atherosclerosis, atheromata—deposits of lipids, calcium, and other material—are the reason artery walls thicken and lose elasticity. In the context of the heart or arteries, atheromata are called atheromatous plaques.

14. See Document 3.4.DiabOver on the DVD.

15. See Document 3.5.DiabFacts on the DVD.

16. Y. Claire Wang et al., "Health and Economic Burden of the Projected Obesity Trends in the USA and the UK," *Lancet* 378:9793 (2011), 815–825, available online at http://www.thelancet.com/journals/lancet/article/PIIS0140-6736(11)60814-3/abstract, September 12, 2012.

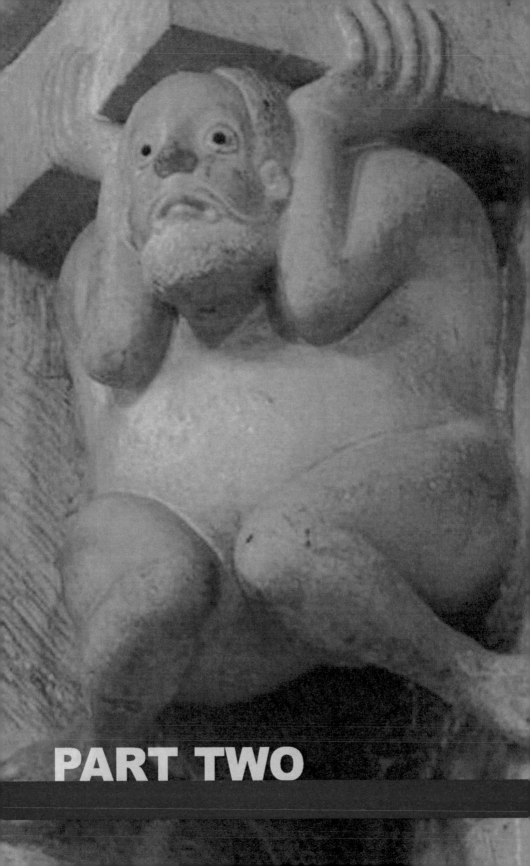

PART TWO

Obesity Treatment

In Part One, we defined what obesity is, why it's reached epidemic proportions, and the health conditions linked to it. In Part Two, we talk about treating obesity.

We begin by outlining the elements that health care providers, patients, and parents of child patients should consider when designing a weight loss program. We then examine the emotional and psychological aspects of weight control, starting with how to avoid eating when you're not truly hungry and ending with strategies to help you to change old habits.

A chapter about calorie requirements and how long it takes to lose excess weight—which includes a great tool for tracking weight loss and lots of resources for healthy cooking—follows. After that, we talk about the part physical activity plays in managing weight and how to get around some common barriers to becoming physically active. Next, we move on to the role of drug and surgical treatments in treating obesity. We conclude by talking about managing weight plateaus and maintaining weight loss for life.

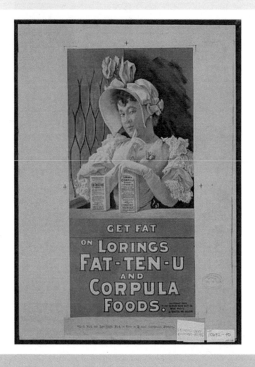

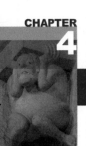

Planning a Weight Loss Program

4

17. What's the health care professional's role in obesity treatment for adults?

For health care providers, treating obesity is a two-phase process. During phase one providers assess the degree to which patients are overweight, their medical histories, lifestyles, and motivation. In this phase, the therapist should consider:

- Medical history, including food sensitivities and allergies
- Family history
- Past history, including illnesses and operations
- Previous efforts to reduce, including failures and successes
- Eating patterns
- Beverage consumption
- Effect of stress and relaxation on eating patterns
- Frequency of eating outside the home
- Sleep patterns, including hours of sleep per night
- Screen time (i.e., time in front of the TV, computer, etc.)
- Physical activity
- Support network
- Cultural beliefs about health and beauty

Phase two consists of managing the weight loss (or weight-maintenance) process. This phase involves developing a treatment plan in consultation with the patient, providing support and helping the patient maintain motivation, and controlling health risks associated with the patient's condition.

For clinical guidelines on treating adults who are overweight or obese, see Document 4.1.ClinGuidelines.

ON THE DVD

Patients deserve respect and empathy from their therapists when discussing their struggles with weight control, and should be encouraged to talk about other issues in their lives that may be interfering with their physical or emotional well-being. Terminology is also important: many overweight people dislike terms such as *fat* and *obese* and instead prefer the more neutral *weight* or *excess weight*, so health care professionals may want to ask patients about their preferences. Lastly, therapists can help patients by working with them to develop realistic treatment plans, by giving practical, specific advice on how much they can eat and how to exercise without injuring themselves, and by recommending products and services that may help.

For advice on talking to patients about losing weight, see Document 4.2.TipsPCPs.

Insofar as possible, obesity treatment plans should conform with the patient's tastes and habits and place limited demands on the family members who are managing the cooking at home. Needless to say, providers of weight loss services need to be honest with patients about the health risks or costs associated with programs, as well as the professional qualifications of themselves and their staff members.

For the *Voluntary Guidelines for Providers of Weight Loss Products or Services* from the Federal Trade Commission (FTC), see Document 4.3.VolGuidelines.

18. What's the health care professional's role in obesity treatment for children?

A health care provider's primary goal should be to prevent a child from becoming overweight in the first place. Not only can long periods of limiting food and increasing activity be difficult for both the child and the therapist, but it's generally much more difficult to treat obesity than to prevent it. Consequently, all children should be screened for overweight and obesity, using BMI percentiles for children older than two years and weight-for-length measurements for younger children. A BMI at or above the 85th percentile and lower than the 95th percentile falls in the overweight range, while a BMI at or above the 95th percentile is considered obese (see Question 9).[1]

For clinical guidelines on screening, preventing, and treating overweight or obese in children and youth, visit:

http://brightfutures.aap.org/pdfs/Guidelines_PDF/5-Promoting_Healthy_Weight.pdf

Children are at a much higher risk for obesity if one or both parents are obese (see Question 7). Those with obese siblings, from low-income families, or with an activity-limiting chronic disease or disability are also at high risk. The child's birth weight, the weight of the mother at the time of delivery, and periods of weight gain (if the child is already overweight) should all be reviewed prior to developing a prevention or treatment plan.

More research is needed to help medical professionals develop obesity prevention and treatment programs for children and adolescents,

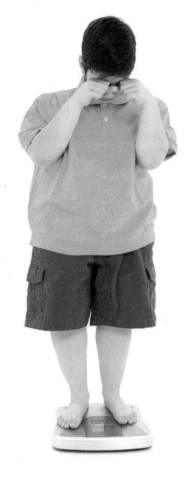

but the process for treating obesity in children is comparable to the one for adults described in Question 17, with some additional considerations. Often weight maintenance—which will result in a gradual decrease in BMI as height increases—is a more appropriate goal for children with no other health issues than weight loss. Rapid weight loss is never healthy for a child.

Therapists need to consider other factors as well when designing a treatment plan for a child. According to the 2007 *Working Group Report on Future Research Directions in Childhood Obesity Prevention and Treatment* from the National Heart, Blood, and Lung Institute (NHBLI), ". . . [d]ifferences in treatment of obesity in youth compared to adults pertain to special circumstances in children's physiology (e.g., growth, pubertal development, fat distribution, comorbidities, side effects from medications), psychosocial factors (e.g., cognitive development, motivating factors, body image, short-term attention span, risk-taking behaviors, lack of concern about health), and environmental influences (e.g., family control, schools, food environment, changing peer groups, effects of advertising, availability of sedentary opportunities). The mainstay of obesity treatment in children and adolescents is to change behaviors related to energy balance. Behavior change in this group is generally safe and, when effective, is generally sustained longer than in adults."[2]

The term **comorbidity**, as used in the 2007 *Working Group Report*, refers to a medical condition related to another medical condition in the same patient. As discussed in Chapter 3, obesity increases the risk of developing diseases such as diabetes and heart disease, two examples of comorbid conditions. Health care professionals must consider comorbidities when choosing a treatment course for obesity.

Meanwhile, an expert committee convened in 2005 by the American Medical Association (AMA), the U.S. Department of Health and Human Services (HHS), and the Centers for Disease Control and Prevention (CDC) recommended a staged treatment approach for overweight and obese children and issued age-specific weight loss guidelines. And the U.S. Preventive Services Task Force (USPSTF) found that intervention programs for children needed to be comprehensive (addressing diet, behavior, and level of physical activity) and of moderate to high intensity (more than 25 hours of contact between the child and/or family and the therapist over a six-month period) to be effective.

For the AMA/HHS/CDC expert committee recommendations, visit:

http://www.ama-assn.org/ama1/pub/upload/mm/433/ped_obesity_recs.pdf

For the USPSTF recommendations, visit:

http://www.uspreventiveservicestaskforce.org/uspstf10/childobes/chobesrs.pdf

19. What role does the patient play in obesity treatment?

Many adults who are overweight start treatment programs on their own, but working with a health care professional can be helpful for the support, expert guidance, and monitoring it offers. (Adults with health issues beyond weight control should definitely consult their health care providers before starting a program.) Whether you work with a therapist or not, remaining positive, motivated, and persistent is extremely important to your success both in weight loss and weight loss maintenance.

For a look at the psychology of weight loss, visit:

http://www.huffingtonpost.com/carole-carson/weight loss-psychology_b_881706.html

For more on the psychology of weight loss, visit:

http://www.livestrong.com/article/167740-psychology-of-weight loss/

For seven strategies to keep you focused on your goals, visit:

http://www.weightwatchers.com/util/art/index_art.aspx?tabnum=1&art_id=48871

Keep in mind that your program is more likely to be successful if:

- It's tailored to your personality and lifestyle
- It sets smaller, incremental goals
- It takes into account your likes and dislikes
- It's sustainable over time

If you're putting a program together yourself, research options—and ask lots of questions if you decide to go to a weight loss clinic (see Document 4.3.VolGuidelines). If you're working with a clinician, you should be developing the program you'll follow

For advice on choosing a weight loss program, see Documents 4.4.ChooseWLProg and 4.5.FindWLProg.

For tips on evaluating weight loss product claims, see Document 4.6.EvalWLProd.

For additional resources on obesity and weight management, see Document 4.7.WeightRes.

together—and again, ask lots of questions. Seeking support from family and friends will help you stay focused once you start your program.

20. What role do parents play in obesity treatment?

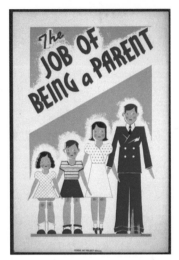

Parents have tremendous influence over the values, attitudes, and habits adopted by family members. One of the most effective things parents can do to help a child maintain a healthy weight is to set a good example with their own eating and exercise patterns. If you think that your child is overweight, your first step should be to consult your health care provider. He or she will be able to tell you whether a gain in weight is part of a developmental phase or an indicator of a weight problem (see also Question 9).

If your child is overweight your health care provider will work with you to develop an appropriate treatment plan, one likely focused on helping your child to grow into his or her weight (see Question 18). There are obvious things you can do to support the plan, such as keeping junk food and sugar-sweetened beverages (which are high in empty calories) out of the house and encouraging daily physical activity.

Junk food is food that is high in calories—often from sugar and fat—but low in nutrition from protein, vitamins, or minerals. Candy, sweet desserts (such as cakes and pies), and salty snacks (such as potato chips and cheese curls) are usually defined as junk food.

DEFINITION

Foods such as hamburgers, tacos, and pizza can be considered junk food depending on how they're prepared and the ingredients used. A small hamburger eaten with vegetables, for example, could be defined as healthy, while a double hamburger with cheese, bacon, and mayonnaise would probably fall into the junk food category due to the large number of calories from fat.

Most of the calories in junk food tend to come from **empty calories**, as calories high in energy and low in nutrients are known. Typical sources are fats, processed carbohydrates (including sugar), and alcohol. According to the NIH, almost 40 percent of calories consumed by young people ages 2–18 comes from empty calories, and half of these are from just six sources: soda, fruit drinks, dairy desserts (ice cream, pudding, custard, etc.), grain-based desserts (cakes, cookies, brownies, etc.), pizza, and whole milk.[3]

There are also some less obvious things that will help:

- Involve the family. Being treated differently makes children feel bad about themselves.

- Don't withhold food. Children may not get the nutrients they need to be healthy, and may learn to sneak food when you're not looking.

- Be supportive and accept children for themselves—at any weight. A positive attitude will help children make the changes they need to.

- Don't use dessert as a reward for eating vegetables. This tells children that vegetables have less value and they'll learn to dislike them.

For more advice on helping your child lose weight, see Documents 4.8.ChildWgtProb and 4.9.HelpOvrwgtChild.

For tips on helping your child eat the right amount, see Document 4.10.ChildAppetite.

21. What strategies are available for obesity treatment?

Treating obesity may take a combination of some or all of the following:

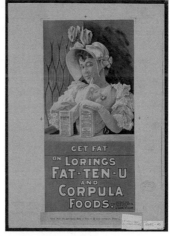

- Dietary therapy

- Physical activity

- Behavior therapy (can include counseling and/or support groups)

- Combined therapy (low-calorie diet, physical activity, behavior therapy)

- Pharmacotherapy, or drug therapy (only to support combined therapy in select patients after six months of combined therapy)

- Weight loss surgery (limited to severely obese patients)

22. What elements should be included in a weight-management program?

Patients, parents of child patients, and health care providers should develop weight loss programs together, and plans must be realistic to be successful. Some of the elements that should be considered when developing a program are:

- Preventing further weight gain. If circumstances preclude creating a plan for weight loss (at least initially), preventing additional weight gain should be an immediate goal.

- Initial weight loss goal.
- Weekly weight loss target.
- Plan for adopting healthy eating habits.
- Plan for adopting healthy physical activity levels.
- Tools for tracking progress.
- Plan for dealing with setbacks and weight plateaus.
- Weight-maintenance plan.
- Cultural needs.

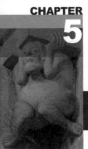

CHAPTER 5

Appetite, Motivation, and Habit

23. What's the difference between hunger and appetite and why is it important?

True **hunger** is motivated by a physiological need for food. It doesn't arise for about 4–6 hours after an adequate meal and generally is accompanied by hunger pangs, a feeling of faintness, and/or a loss of concentration. In contrast, **appetite** is the psychological desire for food. Appetite is stimulated by our thoughts about food, our emotions, proximity to food, and the smell or taste of food.

For seven instances when you should hear *appetite* when your body seems to be saying *hunger*, visit:

ON THE WEB

http://www.time.com/time/photogallery/0,29307,1626481,00.html

For help deciding whether eating more frequently might work for you, visit:

ON THE WEB

http://www.webmd.com/diet/features/truth-about-6-meals-day-weight-loss

To see what experts say about eating three versus six meals a day, visit:

http://www.webmd.com/diet/features/3-hour-diet-or-3-meals-a-day

In the United States and many other developed countries, food is readily available, meaning that we can eat at any time regardless of whether we're hungry. Consequently, managing weight means controlling appetite. We offer strategies for doing this next, but keep in mind that everyone is different, so you'll need to experiment to see what works for you. The idea is to feel full enough throughout the day so that you can stay within your daily caloric budget and only eat in response to true hunger.

Eat more often

Eating six small meals per day helps some people control hunger, food cravings, and blood sugar better than eating three larger ones. You'll need to control portion size based on your daily calorie allowance, and to be satisfying each meal should include lean protein, fiber, and a small amount of healthy fat.

Eat a (healthy!) snack between meals

If your meals are 4–6 hours apart and you find that being overly hungry makes you overeat at mealtime, having a snack between meals can help.

For the art of smart snacking, visit:

http://articles.cnn.com/2007-08-03/health/cl.snacking_1_extra-calories-snacks-mini-meals?_s=PM:HEALTH

Eat breakfast (or not)

Many studies have shown that people who eat breakfast are better at controlling what they eat during the rest of the day and therefore better at maintaining a healthy weight over time. On the other hand, some people feel strongly that if they're not hungry, skipping breakfast allows them to delay their first meal and better control their overall caloric intake. Some experts agree that the second approach can work—for adults, anyway; everyone seems to agree that children do better if they eat breakfast. It all comes down to what helps you stay within your calorie budget.

For the case supporting breakfast, visit:

http://www.webmd.com/diet/features/lose-weight-eat-breakfast

For the case against breakfast, visit:

http://articles.latimes.com/2006/sep/18/health/he-breakfast18

Eat foods high in fiber

Dietary fiber comes from plant foods (meat, milk, and eggs contain no fiber) so eating proportionately more whole grains, legumes, fruits, vegetables, nuts, and seeds will help you increase the fiber in your diet (see Figure 5.1).

▼ FIGURE 5.1
Sources of fiber include whole grains, legumes, fruits, vegetables, nuts, and seeds.

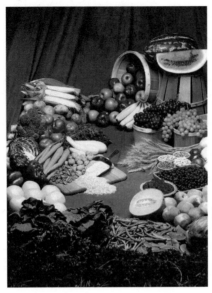

SOURCE: Undated photograph by Keith Weller, Agricultural Research Service, USDA, http://www.ars.usda.gov/is/ graphics/photos/k3839-3.htm

For more on the benefits of fiber, recommendations on how much to eat at each age, and good sources of fiber, visit:

ON THE WEB

http://www.mayoclinic.com/health/ fiber/NU00033

and

http://www.ext.colostate.edu/pubs/ foodnut/09333.html

For tips on adding low-calorie sources of fiber to your diet, visit:

http://www.webmd.com/diet/fiber-health-benefits-11/fiber-weight-control?page=1

For a guide to the fiber content for many foods, see Document 5.1.Fiber.

ON THE DVD

Fiber has many benefits, but with respect to controlling appetite, its advantage lies in its ability to absorb water. This property helps you to feel fuller, longer.

Foods with 5 grams or more per serving are considered **high fiber** by the FDA, those with 2.5–4.9 grams per serving are described as a **good source of fiber**, and those with at least 2.5 grams more per serving than the reference food can be labeled **more fiber** or **added fiber**.

Practice the 20-minute rule

It takes about 20 minutes for your brain to figure out that you're full, and we often don't take this into consideration when we're deciding how much we need to eat.

The first mistake we make is to eat too quickly, which can result in consuming more than our bodies need before our brains tell us we're full. We also help ourselves to seconds before waiting to see if we're really still hungry. Eating slowly and waiting before going for more food will help you to distinguish eating in response to hunger from appetite-driven eating.[4]

Some people find it helpful to write down when they feel the urge to eat—recording the intensity of the urge and whether they ate or not—to better control peak urges not related to hunger. Once they see the patterns and the reasons behind them, they can create strategies that prevent them from eating out of boredom, anxiety, habit, etc.

24. What's the role of the mind in weight loss?

Losing weight and keeping it off requires a change in lifestyle. Committing to big changes necessarily involves altering your thinking, behavior, and beliefs, so understanding the mental adjustments you'll need to make to modify your lifestyle is crucial to maintaining motivation and reaching your goals. We offer three principles to help you adopt a new mind-set next.

For tips to help you avoid eating in response to appetite, visit:

http://www.sparkpeople.com/mypage_public_journal_individual.asp?blog_id=1336070

For a worksheet to record daily craving/eating patterns, see Document 5.2.CraveSheet.

Manage your thinking style/redefine your identity

The National Weight Control Registry (NWCR) is a research study that was started in 1994 to identify and investigate the characteristics of people who have been successful in long-term weight loss.[5] When the NWCR looked at the thinking styles of some of these people, it found that people who were naturally methodical and favored structure and routine had tended to lose the most weight. Fortunately, it's possible to train yourself to become more comfortable with a detail-oriented way of approaching problems—even if you're not naturally inclined to managing details and planning ahead.

Question 19 includes Web links to useful information about the psychology of weight loss.

Another study from the NWCR showed that individuals who were successful with weight loss programs had worked at transforming themselves from within, which allowed them to create a new self that put distance between themselves and old behaviors. This process of redefinition appeared to be critical in maintaining weight loss.

To read about these two NWCR studies (activities to develop a more detail-oriented thinking style are at the end of the article), visit:

http://articles.cnn.com/2007-06-29/living/in.your.head_1_quadrant-national-weight-control-registry-weight loss?_s=PM:LIVING

For success stories from the NWCR, visit:

http://www.nwcr.ws/stories.htm

Deal with negativity

Two steps forward, one step back: setbacks are inevitable when transitioning to a new lifestyle. When you make a mistake, negativity—which adds to stress and may make you more likely to turn a little bump in the road into wholesale abandonment of your goals—is not

For the difference in how optimists and pessimists think, visit:

ON THE WEB

http://www.sparkpeople.com/resource/wellness_articles.asp?id=835

For ways to reframe your conversations with yourself, visit:

ON THE WEB

http://www.centerformedical weightloss.com/health-and-fitness/general-health/channeling-negative-thoughts-into-positive-action/

your friend. Positive thinking really will help you persevere. Beating yourself up won't.

Counteracting negative thoughts first requires paying close attention to how you talk to yourself. Writing down when and how you put yourself down for just a few days (weight loss related or otherwise) will help you see patterns and reframe how you speak to yourself. And changing how you speak to yourself requires practice—just like the lifestyle changes you want to make.

Value mindfulness over willpower

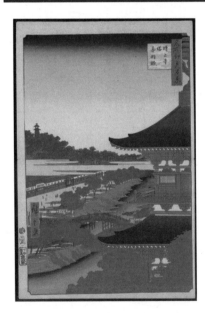

Mindfulness—one of the seven factors of enlightenment in Buddhism—has been incorporated into cognitive behavior therapies by psychotherapists in the West since the 1970s. It has been described as "bringing one's complete attention to the present experience on a moment-to-moment basis."[6] In therapy, practicing mindfulness allows people to become aware of habitual ways of thinking in order to move away from unproductive patterns and respond to life situations in new ways.

Mindfulness is a tool you can use to change your relationship with food. It can help you distinguish appetite from hunger, decrease the amount you eat, gain control of emotional and environmental triggers that cause you to eat when you're not hungry, and enjoy the food you eat more, among other things. It tends to be more effective than using just willpower—which by definition

For more on the benefits and limitations of using mindfulness to change eating behaviors, visit:

ON THE WEB

http://greatergood.berkeley.edu/article/item/better_eating_through_mindfulness

implies inner conflict about the goal and a sense of deprivation—to change behavior, because it allows you to immerse yourself in the act of eating and heighten your enjoyment.

25. Do men and women have different motivations to lose weight?

There are differences between men and women when it comes to losing weight, both in what motivates them and the way they go about it.

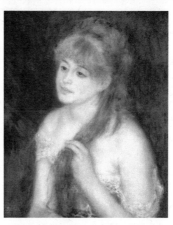

A 2010 Synovate eNation survey conducted on behalf of Herbalife found that women were motivated to lose weight mainly because they were dissatisfied with their appearance, while men cited not feeling healthy as their number one reason. The survey also showed that women were more likely than men to start a weight loss program after gaining only a few pounds, and more likely to try to eat healthier as part of that program. Men and women focused equally on portion control in trying to lose weight, but men were more apt to increase their exercise regimens as part of their programs.[7]

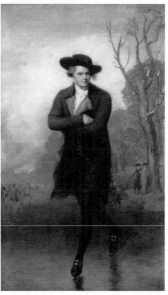

Other data suggests that men are more likely than women to use medical events like heart attacks or advice from doctors as reasons to lose weight, and also are more likely to have realistic weight loss goals. Interestingly, men tend to overeat in response to positive emotions while women overeat in response to negative emotions.[8]

26. How can I change old habits?

A goal without a plan is just a wish. ~ Antoine de Saint-Exupery

When we decide to a pursue a goal that's important to us, such as losing weight, we need to look at eliminating habits that interfere with reaching the goal and cultivating habits that support it. Habits let us perform routine actions without having to think about them too much. These necessary shortcuts are formed by repetition, so it stands to reason that rebuilding behavior patterns also requires practice. Here's a six-step blueprint for changing behavior patterns to achieve your goals.

Define the goal, create a plan

For some advice on setting realistic goals, visit:

http://www.livestrong.com/article/359228-how-to-set-health-goals/

and

http://weightloss.about.com/od/emotionsmotivation/a/aa051707a.htm

Success in changing habits comes from focusing on one habit at a time, breaking required changes into very small, very specific steps, and mastering each step before moving on to the next one. This can feel frustratingly slow, but the science really does support this approach.

Before you can decide which habits do or do not serve you, though, you'll need to define your goals.

So what's your specific weight loss goal? You should choose one that you can reach within six months to a year, because it's harder to stay focused on reaching goals over longer time periods. This may mean that you need to set intermediate weight loss goals.

For example, if you're 5 feet 2 inches tall and weigh 150 pounds, losing 10 percent of your body weight (15 pounds) will put you in the normal range for BMI (see Question 3) and help to lower your risk for heart disease, hypertension, type 2 diabetes, osteoporosis, and certain types of cancer.[9] Since losing 15 pounds in a year or less is achievable for most people, you probably don't need to set an intermediate goal. If, on the other

Question 30 helps you estimate how long it will take to lose excess weight.

hand, you need to lose 30 pounds to get to a normal BMI you probably would want to set an intermediate weight loss goal—maybe 15 pounds.

For elements you should consider in creating your weight loss plan, visit:

http://www.webmd.com/diet/features/plan-day-lose-weight

Once you've decided on the goal you'll need to create a plan with specific steps to get there. This is where you decide which habits you need to change (those that are most likely to undermine or support your efforts) and how you'll prioritize them. For example, a logical first step for your weight loss goal of 15 pounds would be to set a calorie budget—say 2000 calories per day. If you had a habit of eating a couple of small bowls of potato chips in front of the TV at night that might be the first habit you'd want to tackle.

Clarify the reasons for the change

What are your reasons for wanting to lose weight? Not having to worry about developing a serious illness? Wanting to have more energy? Looking better in your clothes? Regardless, your reasons need to be about you (as opposed to pleasing your doctor or spouse) for the incentive to be strong enough to keep you going when you make a mistake or want to give up. The change must be more important to you than the status quo. Many people find it helpful to write their reasons down so they can actually look at them when they need encouragement.

Take stock

Looking at your current eating and exercise patterns will show you what you need to change over time to lose weight. Keeping a food diary for several days will definitely help, because we all tend to underestimate how much and how often we eat, and how little we move.

Start small, be specific

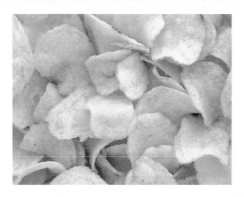

Small, incremental goals give you a chance to practice a new routine. They're also easier to achieve, which will give you confidence and help you take each step in getting to your goal.

Suppose you're working on eliminating the nighttime snacking habit we mentioned earlier. You're full after eating dinner, which means the snacking is driven by appetite, not hunger. The easiest thing to do would be to make sure the chips don't come into the house to begin with, but maybe that's not possible. Here's where you'd outline a series of small steps to retrain yourself. The specific steps should be based on self-awareness: your knowledge of what's driving the habit and the kinds of small steps that might actually help you change it. The speed at which you adopt each subsequent change depends on how long it takes you to master each new step.

For general tips on breaking projects into steps, visit:

http://unclutterer.com/2012/06/14/breaking-projects-down-into-simple-achievable-steps/

For eight specific steps to change any habit, visit:

http://greatergood.berkeley.edu/gg_live/happiness_matters_podcast/podcast/habits_1/

and

http://greatergood.berkeley.edu/gg_live/happiness_matters_podcast/podcast/habits_2/

For tips on combating stress, visit:

http://www.heart.org/HEARTORG/GettingHealthy/StressManagement/FourWaystoDealWithStress/Four-Ways-to-Deal-with-Stress_UCM_307996_Article.jsp

You will most likely have to experiment a bit—which implies failing a bit—to discover what works for you in changing your routine. When you do have setbacks—and you will—resolve to react by telling yourself you'll try something else, rather than giving up.

Prepare yourself for the challenges you might face

The best thing you can do to prepare for challenges is to think ahead. If you're trying to eat no more than 2000 calories per day, for example, think about all the opportunities for overeating that could come up over the course of a day and then figure out ways around them. Be specific—and serious—about how you'll address these roadblocks. Part of thinking ahead is coming up with ways to deal with stress, which often causes our resolve to weaken.

Even if you don't meet all of your goals on a given day you should try to meet at least one of them. If you go over your calorie target for a day, for instance, try to still do any exercise you've planned—it will make you feel better and help you to stay focused and determined. People who engage in efforts to change their behavior and do it for six to eight weeks are more likely to be able to support those efforts long term.

For more on how to create healthy habits, see Document 5.3.CreateHabits and Document 5.4.ChangeHabits.

Track your progress and keep at it

If you can't measure it, you can't manage it.

This principle originated with management consultant, educator, and author Peter Drucker. He was applying it to the world of business, but to meet any kind of goal you need a formal way to track your progress. Many people think they can do this in their heads and don't want to bother with formal tracking systems, but they're indispensable to meeting your goals for the following reasons:

- Your memory isn't as good as you think it is. If you tried to remember what and how much you ate a week ago, could you? Probably not.

- Progress takes time. The incremental changes that happen on a daily basis can go unnoticed or seem inconsequential until you see the cumulative effects.

- You need to focus on the positive. Often we focus on failures and setbacks when we're working toward a goal; tracking systems help you to see all the times you've succeeded, which will help you stay motivated.

- Plans always need tweaking. The plan you start out with will always require adjustments as you go along. Your tracking system will help you to identify what's working for you and what needs rethinking.

- Perspective helps. Tracking systems allow you to see how far you've come and how long results are likely to take.

- A picture paints a thousand words. Tracking systems provide a visual representation of your progress that's very satisfying and will help your resolve.

ON THE WEB

For stories from real people about weight loss strategies that worked for them, visit:

http://www.cdc.gov/healthy weight/success/index.html

Managing Diet CHAPTER 6

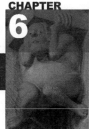

27. What is BMR and what does it have to do with calorie requirements?

Calorie requirements start with the minimum amount of energy needed to keep a body at rest functioning—i.e., fuel for things like respiration, the beating of your heart, and the functioning of other organs. The other basic requirement of calories is for maintenance of body temperature. This minimum amount of calories is known as your **metabolic rate**, **resting metabolic rate (RMR)**, **basal metabolic rate (BMR)**, or simply **metabolism**.[10] About 60–75 percent of calories are expended on BMR.[11] The exact percentage depends on:

- Your size. BMR increases as height and weight increases.
- Your amount of muscle. BMR increases as lean muscle mass increases.

- Your gender. BMR is lower for women than for men of the same size, because women generally have about 10 percent more body fat than men. BMR is higher in pregnant women than in women of the same size who aren't pregnant.

Most factors that affect BMR aren't under our control, but building muscle mass is. A higher proportion of lean tissue will increase BMR, but losing weight still requires controlling calorie intake. There are claims that certain foods and supplements can increase metabolism, but most are unproven.

NOTE

For more on increasing metabolism through lifestyle changes, visit:

http://www.acsm.org/about-acsm/media-room/acsm-in-the-news/2011/08/01/metabolism-is-modifiable-with-the-right-lifestyle-changes

- Your age. BMR is higher in growing children and lower in older people, who usually lose lean muscle mass as they age.
- Individual variation. There does appear to be some unexplained variation in BMR among individuals; research published in the *American Journal of Clinical Nutrition* in 2005 could not explain 26 percent of the variation in BMR among study participants.[12]
- Other factors. Hormonal levels, health issues, and climate also affect BMR.

Diet-induced thermogenesis (heat production through food processing) accounts for about another 10 percent of your body's daily calorie requirements.[13] Food processing includes the digestion, absorption, transportation, and storage of energy from food. Everything you eat is either used for energy or stored for later use.

Physical activity—which includes everything from washing your face to working out at the gym—accounts for the remainder of your calorie requirements (15–30 percent). We'll talk more about its role in promoting health and maintaining weight in Chapter 7.

28. How many calories do I need to maintain my current weight?

As discussed in Question 27, your body's daily calorie expenditure equals BMR + food processing + calories for physical activity. You can get a rough estimate of how many calories you need to maintain your current weight using a formula called the Harris-Benedict equation, originally published as part of a study in 1919 and revised in 1984. The formula consists of two parts: first you calculate BMR calorie requirements (steps 1–3 below), and then you apply a factor to adjust for your activity level (step 4). Here's how the formula works:

1. Measure your height and multiply it by 30.48 to convert it from feet to centimeters. For instance, if you're 5 feet 5 inches tall (5.42 feet tall) you would be $5.42 \times 30.48 = 165.2$ centimeters.

2. Weigh yourself first thing in the morning before you've eaten. Convert your weight from pounds to kilograms by multiplying it by .4536. For instance, if you weigh 150 pounds you would weigh 150 × .4536 = 68.04 kilograms.

3. Estimate your BMR using one of the following formulas, where h = height, w = weight, and a = age.

For men: BMR = [((4.799h + 13.397w) – 5.677a) + 88.362].

For women: BMR = [((3.098h + 9.247w) – 4.330a) + 447.593].

Example 1:

Ted is a 45-year-old man who is 6 feet 3 inches tall (190.5 centimeters) and weighs 230 pounds (104.33 kilograms). His BMR is [((4.799 × 190.5) + (13.397 × 104.33)) – (5.677 × 45)) + 88.362] = 2144.82.

Example 2:

Susan is a 45-year-old woman who is 5 feet 5 inches tall (165.2 centimeters) and weighs 150 pounds (68.04 kilograms). Her BMR is [((3.098 × 165.2) + (9.247 × 68.04)) – (4.330 × 45)) + 447.593] = 1393.7.

4. Multiply your BMR by a factor that reflects your activity level (see Table 6.1).

TABLE 6.1 BMR multipliers for different activity levels

ACTIVITY LEVEL	DESCRIPTION	FACTOR
Sedentary	Little to no daily exercise	1.2
Light activity	Light exercise or sports 1–3 days per week	1.375
Moderate activity	Moderate exercise or sports 3–5 per days per week	1.55
Vigorous activity	Hard exercise or sports 6–7 days per week	1.75
Extra vigorous activity	Very hard exercise or sports in addition to a physical job or physical training two times a day	1.9

SOURCE: J. A. Harris and F. G. Benedict, *A Biometric Study of Basal Metabolism in Man* (Carnegie Institution of Washington: Washington, D.C., 1919).

Assuming a moderate activity level, Ted's required daily calories to maintain his current weight would be BMR × 1.55 = 2144.82 × 1.55 = 3324.47. For Susan, it would be 1393.7 × 1.55 = 2160.24.

Because both Ted and Susan are overweight, the number of calories needed to maintain current weight exceed the number recommended by the 2010 *Dietary Guidelines for Americans* for men and women ages

31–50 who are moderately active: 2400–2600 and 2000, respectively (see Table 6.2).

TABLE 6.2 Estimated calorie needs per day by age, gender, and physical activity level

DAILY CALORIE NEEDS FOR VARIOUS GROUPS				
		PHYSICAL ACTIVITY LEVEL		
Gender	Age (years)	Sedentary	Moderately Active	Active
Child (female and male)	2–3	1000–1200	1000–1400	1000–1400
Female	4–8	1200–1400	1400–1600	1400–1800
	9–13	1400–1600	1600–2000	1800–2200
	14–18	1800	2000	2400
	19–30	1800–2000	2000–2200	2400
	31–50	1800	2000	2200
	51+	1600	1800	2000–2200
Male	4–8	1200–1400	1400–1600	1600–2000
	9–13	1600–2000	1800–2200	2000–2600
	14–18	2000–2400	2400–2800	2800–3200
	19–30	2400–2600	2600–2800	3000
	31–50	2200–2400	2400–2600	2800–3000
	51+	2000–2200	2200–2400	2400–2800

SOURCE: U.S. Department of Agriculture and U.S. Department of Health and Human Services, 2010 *Dietary Guidelines for Americans*, 7th Edition (Washington, D.C.: U.S. Government Printing Office, 2010), 14. See original table for notes (Document 6.1.DietGuide).

Given the number of variables that go into calculating daily calorie needs, you may wonder about the source of the 2000-calorie standard on food labels. The answer is that a benchmark was necessary in order for consumers to be able to see how saturated fat and sodium in foods compared to the FDA's daily allowances, and 2000 calories was both easy to use and close to the recommended daily calories for postmenopausal women, a group particularly vulnerable to weight gain.[14]

You can also estimate your calorie requirements using an online calculator. Remember that calorie calculators, the Harris-Benedict equation, and the USDA guidelines only provide average calorie requirements (for one thing, they don't take proportion of lean muscle mass into consideration), so the numbers they provide may be too high or low for a particular individual, and will most likely differ from each other. Use these kinds of targets as a starting point to estimate your own requirements, and then adjust your levels in small increments based on whether you're gaining, losing, or maintaining weight.

For one of many online calorie calculators, visit:

http://www.acefitness.org/calorie calculators/daily-caloric-needs-calculator.aspx

29. How can I lose weight safely?

Restricting calories too much can make the body think that it's fasting, which tells it to conserve calories and thus interferes with weight loss. Minimum calorie intake varies by body size, age, gender, metabolism, and physical activity level, but the American College of Sports Medicine advises women to eat at least 1200 calories per day and men to eat at least 1800.[15]

For more information on why severe calorie restriction is counterproductive to weight loss, visit:

http://www.livestrong.com/article/548267-long-term-effects-of-dieting-on-resting-metabolic-rate-in-obese-outpatients/

Medical professionals recommend slow, steady weight loss—usually a goal of between one and two pounds per week. Losing weight this way is feasible and safe, and provides time to make and practice necessary lifestyle changes. Moreover, research has shown that people who follow this kind of pattern are more likely to keep weight off over the long term.

The body makes dynamic adjustments in BMR when calorie intake or physical activity levels change. Question 30 discusses how these adjustments affect how long it will take you to lose weight. The SuperTracker tool mentioned in Question 34 will help you calculate a calorie allowance based on your current weight and your goal weight.

An initial goal of 5–10 percent of body weight is realistic and will lower your risk for coronary heart disease and other health problems. For Ted from Question 28, who is 6 feet 3 inches and 230 pounds, that means losing between 12 and 23 pounds. To get to a normal BMI, though, he should weigh 199 pounds or less—a loss of 31 pounds. He therefore should set an initial goal of at least 12 pounds, which will take him about six months (see Question 30). Next he should try to maintain his new weight for six months—if he's successful, he can set a new goal and time frame.

For more on the benefits of losing 10 percent of your body weight, and expert tips on getting there, visit:

http://www.sparkpeople.com/resource/wellness_articles.asp?id=528

30. How long will it take me to lose excess weight?

Weight loss professionals traditionally have advised that a weekly reduction of 3500 calories (500 calories a day) will translate into losing one pound per week. At the same time, there is widespread recognition that the rule—which is based on an estimate that there are 3500 calories 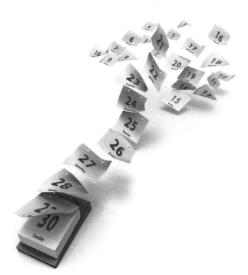 in a pound of fat—is simplistic and will not be representative of most people's experience in losing weight. On the contrary, research has shown that the body continually adjusts both BMR and the number of calories burned during physical activities in response to changes in either calorie intake or activity level. This adjustment means that weight loss will almost certainly take longer than the period projected by the static 3500-calories-equals-one-pound model.

Dr. Kevin Hall and a team of researchers at the NIH have proposed what they consider to be a more accurate rule of thumb, which takes adjustments made by the body into account. Their dynamic model estimates that for the average overweight adult, each permanent reduction of 10 calories per day will result in an eventual loss of a pound, but "with half of the weight change being achieved in about one year and 95 percent of the weight change in about three years."[16]

Both the static and dynamic models project that if you reduce calorie intake permanently by 500 calories a day you can expect to lose a total of about 50 pounds eventually, but they project different time frames to accomplish this. The dynamic model projects that you'll lose 25 pounds after one year (or 25 / 52 weeks = .48 pounds/week) and a total of (50 × .95) = 47.50 pounds after three years. (The .48 pounds per week is an average—weight loss will vary each week not only during the first year but also over the entire course of the weight loss period because of the adjustments your body makes.) In contrast, the static model predicts a steady loss of one pound per week for a total loss of about 52 pounds after one year (see Table 6.3).

TABLE 6.3 Estimated weight loss trajectories under the dynamic and static models

	DYNAMIC MODEL POUNDS LOST	STATIC MODEL POUNDS LOST
3 months	6.23	12.99
6 months	12.47	25.98
9 months	18.70	38.97
12 months	24.94	51.96
36 months	47.50	

SOURCE: Table based on data from Hall et al. (2011), http://www.thelancet.com/journals/lancet/article/PIIS0140-6736(11)60812-x/fulltext

Body composition also impacts how quickly you can lose weight, because body fat stores five times the energy (calories) of muscle. If we accept the estimate that there are 3500 calories in a pound of fat, we can also estimate that there are approximately 700 calories in a pound of muscle. To see the difference, let's assume that weight lost is either all fat or all muscle (which is not the typical pattern). A weekly deficit of 3500 calories—through eating less, exercising more, or a combination of the two—would yield a loss of one pound of fat but five pounds of muscle. In other words, given the same calorie deficit it will take people with more body fat longer to reach a steady-state weight than their leaner counterparts.

Individuals with a high initial percentage of fat will also lose more of their weight in fat relative to lean tissue and lose more weight overall during a given time period than individuals with a higher ratio of muscle. On the other hand, if a calorie surplus is created these individuals will gain more weight than those who are leaner and a larger proportion will be stored as fat.

As weight loss progresses the ratio of fat to muscle changes. As noted in Question 27, BMR increases with muscle mass, but calorie deficits and weight reduction also cause the body to decrease both BMR and the energy cost of a fixed amount of activity, making the precise impact of an increase in muscle mass difficult to gauge. Meanwhile, lean tissue costs the body more energy to build and maintain and contributes more to overall energy expenditures, so as the proportion of muscle increases, the body will have a tendency to preserve energy-rich fat tissue. The bottom line is that as the body becomes leaner, it becomes more and more difficult to lose fat.

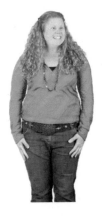

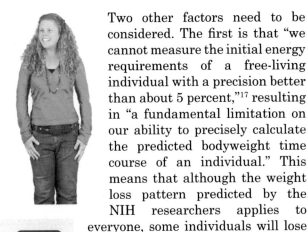

Two other factors need to be considered. The first is that "we cannot measure the initial energy requirements of a free-living individual with a precision better than about 5 percent,"[17] resulting in "a fundamental limitation on our ability to precisely calculate the predicted bodyweight time course of an individual." This means that although the weight loss pattern predicted by the NIH researchers applies to everyone, some individuals will lose weight a little more quickly and some a little more slowly because of the uncertainty of determining how many calories a given person needs to maintain his or her baseline weight. Also, it appears that activity level itself has a more complicated impact on weight gain, maintenance, and loss than was perhaps previously appreciated.

For more on the NIH study and its implications, visit:

http://www.nytimes.com/2011/09/20/health/20brody.html?pagewanted=all&_r=0

ON THE WEB

Given the many variables at work, it can be hard to estimate how long it will take to see results from a weight loss program. Dr. Hall and his colleagues have developed the Web-based Body Weight Simulator to help with this, which shows the time necessary to reach a goal weight under different scenarios. Their application calculates estimated baseline calories based on height, weight, age, gender, and activity level. You can then enter a goal weight and a time frame for achieving that weight, and the application will show you the calorie reduction needed and graph how weight loss will progress over that period. Users can also specify lifestyle changes to see how they impact results.

To use the Body Weight Simulator, visit:

http://bwsimulator.niddk.nih.gov/

TOOLS

31. What is healthy eating?

In a nutshell, healthy eating patterns allow individuals to get the nutrients they need to promote health while maintaining a weight appropriate for their height. Research supports a diet that emphasizes vegetables and fruits (which have a high vitamin, mineral, and fiber content); whole grains (which are rich in fiber, minerals, and vitamins); moderate amounts of lean protein, including protein from plant-based sources (to provide minerals and to help the body build and repair tissue); and monounsaturated instead of saturated fats.

Healthy diets also limit intake of sodium and added sugars and control portion sizes.

There are many free online resources that provide advice on healthy eating, including those provided by the U.S. Department of Agriculture (USDA), the U.S. Department of Health and Human Services (HHS), the Centers for Disease Control and Prevention (CDC), and the National Institutes for Health (NIH). The USDA has been providing nutrition advice to Americans since 1894, and over time both its recommendations and the format in which they're offered has evolved. In 2011, MyPlate became the USDA's new nutritional guide (see Figure 6.1).

It replaced MyPryamid, a 2005 redesign of an earlier food pyramid (see Figure 6.2).

The original Food Guide Pyramid was introduced in 1992 (see Figure 6.3).

▼ FIGURE 6.1
2011 MyPlate graphic.

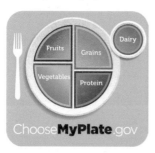

SOURCE: U.S. Department of Agriculture, http://www.ChooseMyPlate.gov/print-materials-ordering/graphic-resources.html

▼ FIGURE 6.2
2005 MyPyramid graphic.

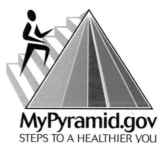

SOURCE: U.S. Department of Agriculture, http://www.ChooseMyPlate.gov/print-materials-ordering/graphic-resources.html

▼ FIGURE 6.3
1992 Food Guide Pyramid graphic.

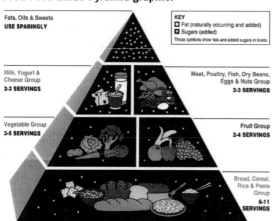

SOURCE: U.S. Department of Agriculture, http://www.cnpp.usda.gov/FGPGraphicResources.htm

For plate versus pyramid guidelines, visit:

http://www.sparkpeople.com/resource/nutrition_articles.asp?id=425

ON THE WEB

MyPlate is based on the 2010 *Dietary Guidelines for Americans* (guidelines will be updated in 2015) that's produced jointly by HHS and the USDA. Many experts, including those at the American Heart Association and the Academy of Nutrition and Dietetics, consider MyPlate to be a big improvement over the pyramid, both in terms of presentation and guidelines.

The new MyPlate graphic is meant to show what a filled, nine-inch plate should look like: roughly one-half fruits and vegetables, one-quarter grains (preferably whole grains), and one-quarter protein. There's a small circle to the side of the plate to represent low-fat dairy products. In contrast, the pyramid emphasized required daily servings from each of five food groups (plus one for fats, oils, and sweets), which meant that consumers needed to add up servings throughout the day to see if they were meeting daily requirements. The ChooseMyPlate Web site has a variety of resources and tools to help users eat a balanced diet and manage weight.

To check out the new ChooseMyPlate Web site, visit:

http://www.choosemyplate.gov/

For information on the five food groups, visit:

http://www.choosemyplate.gov/food-groups/

ON THE WEB

For comments on the switch to MyPlate from a variety of health professionals and organizations, visit:

http://www.foodpolitics.com/2011/06/everybody-loves-myplate-really/

ON THE WEB

MyPlate's emphasis on fruits and vegetables is also new, and supported even by those who feel that its recommendations still need more work. Among the criticisms is that dairy products (a source of protein) should be included in the protein quadrant, and that a separate protein section may be unnecessary to begin with because grains and legumes (the latter are part of the vegetable section) are also important sources of protein. By not addressing fats at all (which are necessary for good health), MyPlate also fails to help consumers choose those that are healthier. Critics of the new symbol also point out the disconnect between the MyPlate recommendations and what U.S. agricultural subsidies actually support.

To review the 2010 *Dietary Guidelines for Americans*, see Document 6.1.DietGuide.

For a brochure and the *Ten Tips* series of tip sheets that summarize key recommendations from the 2010 guidelines, see Documents 6.1.1.DGTips through 6.1.24.TTSafety.

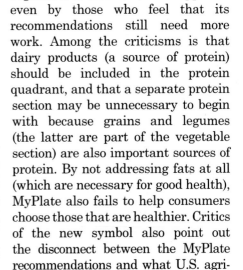

ON THE DVD

Notwithstanding the criticism, dietary recommendations from countries around the world are fairly consistent with MyPlate's guidelines, so on the whole they're a good jumping-off point (although you'll probably find that you'll need to supplement information on the MyPlate site with other resources).

32. What's the difference between a serving size and a portion?

The **serving size** that you see on nutrition labels is based on typical portion sizes as determined by food consumption surveys. A **portion** is the amount of food you put on your plate. Eating portion sizes that are larger than what is considered typical is one of the main contributors to overweight and obesity, so it's important to be familiar with recommended serving sizes for different foods and what they look like.

For a guide to recommended serving sizes and visual comparisons to common objects, see Documents 6.2.FoodAmt and 6.3.SrvSize.

For tips on portion control, see Document 6.4.PortionCtrl.

33. How do I read a nutrition label?

Nutrition labels are important because they let you know how a food fits into your daily budget for calories, fat, and nutrients—but the amount of information they contain can make them confusing to read.

It helps to understand that the label is composed of different sections, each of which provides you with a different kind of information (see Figure 6.4).

Nutrition labels can also help you to distinguish between commonly used—but similar sounding—food terms, such as low fat and reduced fat.

For information on how to use nutrition labels to meet your dietary needs, visit:

http://www.youtube.com/watch?v=Hg6ru8XatGo&list=LPze3_X4IKgmQ&index=4&feature=plcp

In deciding whether a food meets your dietary needs, the 5/20 rule can help too: foods that contain 5 percent or less of the recommended daily value (DV) of a nutrient aren't a good source of the nutrient, while foods that contain 20 percent or more are.

For example, if you're trying to increase fiber in your diet (which helps you to feel more full and eat less—see Question 23), you'd look for foods that contain at least 20 percent of DV for fiber. Conversely, to limit fat, cholesterol, and sodium intake you'd look for foods with less than 5 percent of the DV.

Nutrition Facts

Serving Size 1 cup (228g)
Servings Per Container 2

Amount Per Serving

Calories 250   Calories from Fat 110

	% Daily Value*
Total Fat 12g	18%
Saturated Fat 3g	15%
Trans Fat 3g	
Cholesterol 30mg	10%
Sodium 470mg	20%
Potassium 700mg	20%
Total Carbohydrate 31g	10%
Dietary Fiber 0g	0%
Sugars 5g	
Protein 5g	
Vitamin A	4%
Vitamin C	2%
Calcium	20%
Iron	4%

* Percent Daily Values are based on a 2,000 calorie diet.
Your Daily Values may be higher or lower depending on
your calorie needs.

	Calories:	2,000	2,500
Total Fat	Less than	65g	80g
Sat Fat	Less than	20g	25g
Cholesterol	Less than	300mg	300mg
Sodium	Less than	2,400mg	2,400mg
Total Carbohydrate		300g	375g
Dietary Fiber		25g	30g

Start here

Check calories

Quick guide to % DV

5% or less is low
20% or more is high

Limit these

Get enough of these

Footnote

SOURCE: Health.gov, http://www.health.gov/Dietaryguidelines/dga2005/
toolkit/Worksheets/foodlabel.htm

34. How can I manage my diet to lose weight?

Improving how you manage your weight starts with figuring out what
you and your family consume, then determining how many calories you
should be consuming and the mix of nutrients you need for a balanced
diet. You'll also need to look at your physical activity level to see if you
need to become more active: most Americans aren't active enough.

Next you'll need a tracking system to establish your baseline and monitor your progress (see Question 26). You'll want to pick a tool that you're comfortable using that also lets you track calories and activity accurately

For the FDA's guide to using nutrition labels to make healthy food choices, see Document 6.5.NutLabelGuide.

and consistently. ChooseMyPlate offers a tool called SuperTracker that lets you set up a personalized plan and has features that allow you to compare what you eat to nutrition targets, track your physical activity and your weight, get coaching help, and run a variety of reports. You can also share your results on Facebook and Twitter.

SuperTracker has its limitations, of course. For example, some foods can be hard to find because of the way they're listed, and while the database of foods is relatively large it's far from complete. They've just added a feature that allows you to customize food items, however, and you can also submit requests to add foods. Despite any drawbacks, SuperTracker is a far easier and more convenient tracking method than pen and paper (a mobile app is in the works). If you find it's not a good fit for you, though, an online

To use SuperTracker, visit:

https://www.Supertracker.usda.gov/

For two other online tracking systems, visit:

http://www.fitbit.com/

and

http://www.myfitnesspal.com/

For a guide to using SuperTracker, see Document 6.6.SuprTrkrGuide.

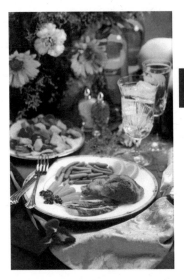

search will lead you to plenty of others in addition to the alternatives we've already listed.

35. How can I make my tracking system work for me?

Remembering what you ate, figuring out portion sizes, and decoding what's in a restaurant dish are three common problems with keeping track of what you're eating. At the same time, tracking calories won't help you reach your goal unless the information you record is accurate. Getting around these obstacles—and whatever others come up—is the key to making a tracking system work for you.

Remembering what you ate

For a basic weekly worksheet to track food and activity, see Document 6.7.FoodActLog.

ON THE DVD

For a basic daily worksheet that will help you identify emotional eating, see Document 6.8.FoodFeelLog.

To download daily food-tracking worksheets that are customized for your calorie level and include tips on serving sizes and food groups, visit:

ON THE WEB

http://www.choosemyplate.gov/professionals/food_tracking_wksht.html

Entering your meals in an online system right after you eat should be relatively easy if you have un-interrupted Internet access, but otherwise you can use food-tracking worksheets or a journal as stopgaps until you can enter the information. Worksheets don't need to be very detailed: all that's needed is space to jot down notes.

Some people prefer worksheets that remind them of their goals. The old MyPyramid worksheets provide basic portion and nutrient guidelines, along with an area to record daily physical activity.

Figuring out portion sizes

To find out how to use your hand to estimate portion sizes, visit:

http://www.youtube.com/watch?v=CA-wyKqKjpI
ON THE WEB

Sometimes it can be hard to translate what you see on your plate into ounces or cups. Documents 6.2.FoodAmt and 6.3.SrvSize (referenced in Question 32) can help you with this. Also, the Food Groups section of the

ChooseMyPlate Web site includes galleries for each food group that show what serving sizes look like (see Question 31). You can also use your hand—just click the On the Web link for a video demonstration.

Decoding what's in a restaurant dish

Identifying ingredients and nutrients in dishes can be challenging if you're eating out. In many restaurants, your server will know (or can find out) what's in a menu item: specialized dietary requirements and food allergies mean that these questions are not out of the ordinary these days. Restaurants often post nutrition information on their Web sites as well, and there are a number of Web sites that post calorie and nutrient information for menu items at different chain restaurants. If a restaurant can't or won't share this information, though, your best bet may be to choose another place.

To check calorie counts and nutritional information for menu items at a variety of chain restaurants, visit:

http://caloriecount.about.com/restaurants-mc1?s_order=a
or

http://www.nutritionix.com/

(These sites include calorie counts for other food product categories too.)

36. Where can I find calorie and nutrition information for different foods?

SuperTracker's Food-A-Pedia gets its calorie and nutrition information from the USDA database, which has profiles for more than 8,000 foods. There are many other online options as well (two are referenced in Question 35).

To access the USDA database, visit:

http://ndb.nal.usda.gov/

To use the food and nutrition browsers from the Calorie Count Web site, visit:

http://caloriecount.about.com/foods

37. What are your top five tips for reducing calories?

Here are five solid tips for reducing your calorie intake (you should also review Chapter 5, which discusses different strategies to help you avoid overeating):

- Drink water instead of alcohol, soda, and other sugary drinks.
- Don't bring junk food into the home.
- Cook at home whenever possible—it's cheaper, and it will allow you to control portion sizes, nutrients, sodium, sugar, and the fat content of your meals better.

For 25 more tips on reducing calories, visit:

http://usatoday30.usatoday.com/yourlife/fitness/weight loss-challenge/2011-01-03-WLCbesttips03_ST_N.htm

ON THE WEB

For tips on cooking at home more, visit:

http://www.choosemyplate.gov/weight-management-calories/weight-management/better-choices/cook-home.html

For green smoothie recipes, visit:

http://www.rawfamily.com/recipes

For four tips to help your child manage his or her weight, visit:

http://www.uctv.tv/shows/The-Skinny-on-Obesity-Extra-Four-Sweet-Tips-from-Dr-Lustig-23901

- Try green smoothies if you can't seem to eat enough fruits and vegetables.
- Use nonfood rewards to cope with stress.

38. What are your top five tips for healthy eating on a budget?

Healthy food has the reputation of costing more than junk food, but it really depends on how you measure price. Studies traditionally have used a per-calorie metric, which tends to give energy-dense junk food the edge over healthier options. If you measure on the basis of edible weight or average portion size, though, "grains, vegetables, fruit, and dairy foods are less expensive than most protein foods and foods high in saturated fat, added sugars, and/or sodium."[19] Here are some tips for eating well on a budget:

- Spend an hour planning the week's meals on the weekend, make a shopping list, and stick to it.
- Buy seasonal, reduced-price, or frozen produce.
- Buy whole foods instead of processed ones.

For other tips on spending less to eat well, see Document 6.9.BudgetEats.

For a weekly meal planner, see Document 6.10.MealPlan.

ON THE DVD

- Plan a couple of meals a week that use legumes instead of meat for protein.
- Buy nonperishable foods in bulk, and perishable foods in small amounts.

For the basics of meal planning, visit:

http://foodformyfamily.com/the-kitchen-sink/eat-well-spend-less-menus-and-meal-planning

and

http://wellnessmama.com/5345/7-meal-planning-basics/

ON THE WEB

Sometimes beginning cooks (or even those who have fallen out of practice) find meal planning intimidating, but it doesn't take long to get the hang of it. Planning helps you to use one food for more than one meal in different ways and to use your leftovers (including leftover perishable items that are hanging around) so that you save time and money.

39. What are your top five tips for healthy eating outside the home?

Sticking to a weight loss plan can be challenging when you eat out, whether at a restaurant or a dinner party: it's harder to control what's on your plate and there's a temptation to think of a meal out as an opportunity to treat yourself (see Question 35). A 2011 survey found that the average American eats 4.8 meals a week in a restaurant, though, so sticking to a weight loss program requires discipline inside and outside the home.[20] Here are five tips for staying on the straight and narrow when you're eating out:

* Review the menu online and choose your meal before you go.
* Skip the bread or limit yourself to a small piece—preferably without butter or oil.
* Have a cup of low-fat soup or a small salad (dressing on the side) as a starter to help you eat less of your entree.
* Request a take-home container when you order and put half your meal in it before you start eating.
* Don't hesitate to ask for modifications—sauce on the side, no fries—or even order off the menu to get what you want.

 For a pocket guide to healthy eating on the go, see Document 6.11.HthyWgtOnGo.

40. How about some healthy recipe suggestions?

There are lots of sites with healthy recipes—an online keyword search of *healthy recipes* returns millions of results.

SuperTracker is one of these sources: it has meal templates that show you how to combine meals and snacks to meet daily food group targets, with drop-down screens that list foods for each group. The USDA also offers a recipe finder that includes nutrition and cost information and comes with a feature that lets you build your own cookbook. And some sites offer cooking videos to make things even easier. Check out the links that follow for a sampling of sites with healthy recipes.

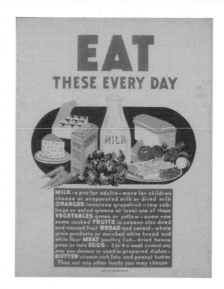

The DVD also has resources on healthy eating and meal planning, as well as a general guide to managing weight.

To build meals tailored to your needs using SuperTracker's Sample Meal Plans feature, visit:

https://www.SuperTracker.usda.gov/samplemealplans.aspx

To use the USDA's recipe finder and/or create your own cookbook, visit:

http://recipefinder.nal.usda.gov/cookbook

To search for recipes by special diet or ingredient at the Mayo Clinic site, visit:

http://www.mayoclinic.com/health/healthy-recipes/RecipeIndex

For videos that show you how to prepare low-calorie recipes and make a number of recipes healthier, visit:

http://recipes.sparkpeople.com/videos-home.asp

and

http://hp2010.nhlbihin.net/healthyeating/Video.aspx

For other healthy recipes, visit Crestor's site at:

http://www.crestor.com/c/mealplanner/home.aspx

and

http://www.crestor.com/c/your-arteries/living-healthy/eating-healthy-diet/food-university.aspx

For a number of other online resources, visit:

http://www.cdc.gov/healthyweight/healthy_eating/recipes.html

For guidance on using fruits and vegetables to manage your weight, see Document 6.12.HthyWgtFV and Document 6.13.UseFVWgt.

For flavorful, low-calorie recipes, see Document 6.14.Dinners.

For healthy recipes for the whole family, see Document 6.15.FamMeals.

For a comprehensive guide to weight management that provides tips on low-fat cooking methods and decreasing fat and calories in your diet, samples of reduced-calorie meals and ways to stay on track when you eat out, and information about increasing your physical activity, see Document 6.16.AimHthyWgt.

Managing Activity

CHAPTER 7

41. What's the difference between physical activity and exercise?

Technology and lifestyle changes in industrialized countries have made it easy to avoid not only exercise but even a healthy level of routine physical activity. Both are different kinds of **physical activity**, which covers anything from brushing your teeth to washing dishes to running a marathon—basically, any movement that requires you to contract your muscles and use energy in excess of BMR.

A **routine physical activity** is a low-intensity life activity—such as vacuuming, walking around the supermarket, and folding laundry—that causes you to move around but doesn't require a lot of effort. **Exercise**, on the other hand, is physical exertion that lasts long enough and is hard enough to help you become healthier and more physically fit. We usually think of things like bicycling, sit-ups, or swimming when we think of exercise, but playing Frisbee, ballroom dancing, and planting shrubs can count as exercise too. The key is intensity: for example, strolling would be a routine physical activity for most people, while walking briskly would count as exercise for almost everyone.

Throughout this chapter we'll use the terms *physical activity* and *exercise* more or less interchangeably, just as most people do. If we're talking about just routine physical activity or exercise we'll make that clear.

Most people who are active through-out the day because of their jobs (construction workers, nurses, park rangers, etc.) or lifestyles (for example, people who run after a child all day,

NOTE

There seems to be no universally accepted definition of **physical fitness**, but many experts agree that there are five components: cardiovascular endurance, muscle strength, muscle endurance, flexibility, and body composition. A health club professional can perform tests to assess where you stand with respect to each of these components and create a personalized exercise program based on the results. For more information on each component, visit:

http://www.fitday.com/fitness-articles/
fitness/body-building/the-5-components-of-
physical-fitness.html#b

ON THE WEB

For research findings on how too much sitting can promote weight gain, interfere with body processes, and increase the risk of developing certain health conditions, visit:

http://www.nytimes.com/2011/04/17/
magazine/mag-17sitting-t.html?_r=0

For tips on using routine physical activity to help manage your weight, visit:

http://usatoday30.usatoday.com/news/health/
weightloss/2009-01-21-fidget-activity_N.htm

do many of their errands on foot, or have hobbies like gardening) still need to exercise, because their daily activities are not usually intense and varied enough to bestow physical fitness.

Conversely, people who exercise still need to be physically active throughout the day. For one thing, routine physical activity helps burn calories. (The new field of inactivity research even suggests that habitual low levels of activity may be the difference between those who don't gain weight and those who do.) For another, a number of studies show that too much sitting can increase the risk for serious health conditions and a shortened lifespan.

42. What is the role of physical activity in weight control?

Research has suggested for a long time that physical activity is an essential part of weight control, but exactly how it helps the body maintain energy balance is still not well understood. As James Hill and Holly Wyatt at the Center for Human Nutrition at the University of Colorado Denver (and also the National Weight Control Registry— see Question 24) put it, "[t]here is very little argument about the states of energy balance or imbalance that produce weight gain, weight loss, or weight stability, but there is considerable argument about the respective roles of diet and physical activity in achieving each of these energy balance goals."[21]

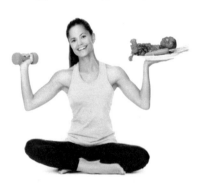

Experts agree on some things, though. There seems to be consensus, for example, that although physical activity alone won't help you lose weight, it's critical in maintaining weight loss—even if we aren't yet sure exactly why. Studies (some of which goes back a number of decades) also indicate that weight gain is all but inevitable below a certain threshold of physical activity. For example, in a study published in 1956 of 213 mill workers in West Bengal, India, whose jobs covered a wide range of physical activity (sedentary to very physical work), "[i]t was found that calorie intake increases with activity only within a certain zone ("normal activity"). Below that range ("sedentary zone") a decrease in activity is not accompanied by a decrease in food intake, but, on the contrary, by an increase. Body weight is also increased in that zone."[22]

These results were consistent with those of another study published in 1956 that followed obese high school girls in the Boston suburbs, which found that the average calorie intake of the overweight girls was the same as normal-weight girls of similar age, height, and grade, but that their activity level was far less.[23] They're also generally supported by data from more recent research.[24] The West Bengal study concluded that "[t]he fact that mechanized, urbanized modern living may well be pushing an ever greater fraction of the population into the "sedentary" range may thus be a major factor in the increased incidence of obesity."[25]

For recent research results on the relationship between physical activity, appetite, and weight management, visit:

http://www.nytimes.com/2010/04/18/magazine/18exercise-t.html?pagewanted=all&_r=1&

There's also agreement that it's easier to gain weight than to lose it, as a result of how the body's energy balance system is calibrated. (This is on top of the issue of metabolic imbalance at low activity levels just discussed.) Consequently, preventing (or at least limiting) weight gain when possible is an "easier" route to maintaining a healthy weight. As James Hill, Holly Wyatt, and John Peters comment in a study published in 2012, "[m]atching energy intake to a high level of energy expenditure will likely be more feasible for most people than restricting food intake to meet a low level of energy expenditure. Second, from an energy balance point of view, we are likely to be more successful in preventing excessive weight gain than in treating obesity. The reason is that the energy balance system shows stronger opposition to weight loss than to weight gain. Although large behavior changes are needed to produce and maintain reductions in body weight, small behavior changes may be sufficient to prevent excessive weight gain. The concept of energy balance combined with an understanding of how the body achieves balance may be a useful framework for developing strategies to reduce obesity rates."[26]

See Question 30 for some background on how the body's energy balance system adjusts in response to changes in calorie intake and/or physical activity levels.

Other research findings indicate that the body seems to be able to regulate energy balance better with a certain (high) level of physical activity. This is possibly because of evolutionary advantage, according to Hill, Wyatt, and Peters, who write, "[o]n the basis of our review

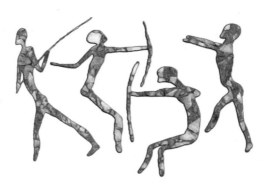

of the energy balance literature and information about how our modern lifestyle differs from decades ago, we hypothesize that human physiology developed under circumstances that conferred an advantage for achieving energy balance at a relatively high (compared with RMR) level of energy expenditure—a high energy throughput—or high energy flux.[27]

Two final notes. First, it appears that even with sufficient levels of physical activity women may have a harder time losing weight than men—primarily because they carry about 10 percent more body fat (see Question 3), but also because unlike men, exercise may increase levels of the hunger hormone ghrelin (see On the Web on this page). Other factors that may make it harder for women to lose weight may be at work as well.

For a look at the factors that may make it harder for women to lose weight, visit:

ON THE WEB

http://ideas.time.com/2012/07/03/double-standard-women-must-work-harder-to-lose-weight/

Second, it's critical for children to be active—for normal-weight children because of activity's role in helping to prevent weight gain, for overweight children who are growing because it will likely reduce the need for dietary restrictions in a weight loss program, and for all children because it will help lay a foundation for a lifetime of regular physical activity.

43. What are the four main types of physical activity and what are the benefits of each?

The four main types of physical activity are aerobic, muscle-strengthening, bone-strengthening, and stretching.

Aerobic activity (also referred to as **cardiovascular activity, cardio,** or **endurance activity**) increases your heartbeat and will make your heart and lungs stronger if you do it regularly. It also helps your stamina and improves your circulation. During aerobic activities you use your large muscle groups (such as those in your arms and legs). Examples include running, walking, swimming, dancing, and bicycling.

For a video database of cardio exercises, visit:

ON THE WEB

http://www.bodybuilding.com/exercises/finder/lookup/filter/exercisetype/id/2/

Muscle-strengthening activity and **bone-strengthening activity** are both types of **strength training,** which is also known as **weight training.** Muscle-strengthening activities increase the strength, power, and endurance of your muscles. When you do bone-strengthening activities your arms, legs, or feet support your weight and your muscles press against your bones.

Many activities help both your muscles and your bones, and if the activity makes your heart and lungs work harder it can be aerobic as well. Lifting free weights, using weight machines, and doing push-ups are examples of activities that strengthen both your muscles and your bones. Running, walking, and dancing are endurance activities that will also help bones and muscles. Activities like swimming and bicycling are good for your cardiovascular system, but depending on the intensity at which they're performed can be less effective for strengthening bones and muscles because your body is supported while you do them.

For a video database of strength-training exercises, visit:

http://www.bodybuilding.com/exercises/finder/lookup/filter/exercisetype/id/1/

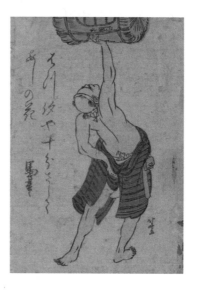

Stretching is the fourth type of physical activity. Stretching helps you improve flexibility, prevent muscle injury, and retain a full range of movement in your joints. It also helps your body warm up and prepare for endurance or weight training. Simple movements such as circling your arms, touching your toes, and lunges are all examples of activities that increase your flexibility. Practicing yoga on a regular basis is an excellent way to build flexibility while strengthening muscles and bones.

In addition to the four main types of activities, there is a fifth: activities that help your balance. **Balance activities** are good for everyone, but they're particularly important for older people because they can help prevent falls that may result in bone fractures. Any activity that requires you to be on your feet and moving— such as walking—will help balance. You can also practice standing on

For a video database of stretching exercises, visit:

http://www.bodybuilding.com/exercises/finder/lookup/filter/exercisetype/id/3/

For a five-part yoga video series aimed at beginners, visit:

http://www.youtube.com/playlist?list=PL68C4F42A875FF6B0

To see a video demonstration of three balancing exercises for beginners, visit:

http://www.youtube.com/watch?v=5N0u5d6RZT4

For a video showing a wider variety of balance exercises, visit:

http://www.youtube.com/watch?v=AWuKEt96Jjs

ON THE WEB

one foot, standing on your tiptoes, and getting in and out of a chair without using your arms for support to improve your balance.

44. How much exercise do I need?

In 2008, the U.S. government issued its first comprehensive guidelines on physical activity, which came out of an extensive review of the scientific literature on the subject. The guidelines are consistent with recommendations from the American Heart Association and the American College of Sports Medicine.

Physical Activity Guidelines for Americans is intended to complement *Dietary Guidelines for Americans* (see Question 31 and Document 6.1.DietGuide), and provides recommended activity levels for Americans age six and older. There are also key guidelines for six subgroups—children and adolescents (those ages 6–17), adults (those ages 18–64), older adults (those age 65 and older), adults with disabilities, women during pregnancy and the postpartum period, and people with chronic medical conditions. We'll outline what those are next.[28]

Children and adolescents

- Children and adolescents should do 60 minutes (1 hour) or more of physical activity daily.

- Aerobic: Most of the 60 or more minutes a day should be either moderate- or vigorous-intensity aerobic physical activity, and should include vigorous-intensity physical activity at least three days a week.

- Muscle-strengthening: As part of their 60 or more minutes of daily physical activity, children and adolescents should include muscle-strengthening physical activity on at least three days of the week.

- Bone-strengthening: As part of their 60 or more minutes of daily physical activity, children and adolescents should include bone-strengthening physical activity on at least three days of the week.

- It is important to encourage young people to participate in physical activities that are appropriate for their age, that are enjoyable, and that offer variety.

- All adults should avoid inactivity. Some physical activity is better than none, and adults who participate in any amount of physical activity gain some health benefits.

- For substantial health benefits, adults should do at least 150 minutes (2 hours and 30 minutes) a week of moderate-intensity aerobic physical activity, or 75 minutes (1 hour and 15 minutes) a week of vigorous-intensity aerobic physical activity, or an equivalent combination of moderate- and vigorous-intensity aerobic activity. Aerobic activity should be performed in episodes of at least 10 minutes and preferably spread throughout the week.

- For additional and more extensive health benefits, adults should increase their aerobic physical activity to 300 minutes (5 hours) a week of moderate-intensity aerobic physical activity, or 150 minutes a week of vigorous-intensity aerobic physical activity, or an equivalent combination of moderate- and vigorous-intensity activity. Additional health benefits are gained by engaging in physical activity beyond this amount.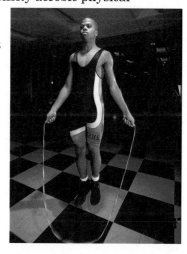

- Adults should also do muscle-strengthening activities that are moderate or high intensity and involve all major muscle groups on two or more days a week, as these activities provide additional health benefits.

Older adults (supplement to adult guidelines)

- When older adults cannot do 150 minutes of moderate-intensity aerobic activity a week because of chronic conditions, they should be as physically active as their abilities and conditions allow.

- Older adults should do exercises that maintain or improve balance if they are at risk of falling.

- Older adults should determine their level of effort for physical activity relative to their level of fitness.

- Older adults with chronic conditions should understand whether and how their conditions affect their ability to do regular physical activity safely.

Adults with disabilities

- Adults with disabilities should get at least 150 minutes a week of moderate-intensity or 75 minutes a week of vigorous-intensity aerobic activity or an equivalent combination of moderate- and vigorous-intensity aerobic activity if they're able to. Aerobic activity should be performed in episodes of at least 10 minutes and preferably spread throughout the week.

- Adults with disabilities should also do muscle-strengthening activities of moderate or high intensity that involve all major muscle groups on two or more days a week if they're able to, as these activities provide additional health benefits.

- When adults with disabilities are not able to meet these guidelines, they should engage in regular physical activity according to their abilities and should avoid inactivity.

- Adults with disabilities should consult their health care providers about the amounts and types of physical activity that are appropriate for their abilities.

Women during pregnancy and the postpartum period

- Healthy women who are not already highly active or doing vigorous-intensity activity should get at least 150 minutes of moderate-intensity aerobic activity a week during pregnancy and the postpartum period. This activity preferably should be spread throughout the week.

- Pregnant women who habitually engage in vigorous-intensity aerobic activity or who are highly active can continue physical activity during pregnancy and the postpartum period, provided that they remain healthy and discuss with their health care providers how and when activity should be adjusted over time.

People with chronic medical conditions

- Adults with chronic conditions obtain important health benefits from regular physical activity.

- When adults with chronic conditions do activity according to their abilities, physical activity is safe.

- Adults with chronic conditions should be under the care of a health care provider. People with chronic conditions and symptoms should consult their health care providers about the types and amounts of activity appropriate for them.

Physical Activity Guidelines for Americans also includes information on how the guidelines were formulated, the health benefits of physical

ON THE DVD

To review the 2008 *Physical Activity Guidelines for Americans*, see Document 7.1.PAGuide.

If you're an adult, get help on starting, maintaining, and increasing the intensity of a physical activity program from Document 7.2.AdultGuide.

To see how exercise can help your heart, and for tips on starting a physical fitness program, see Document 7.3.PAHeart.

For a quick summary that hits the highlights of *Physical Activity Guidelines for Americans*, see Document 7.4.PAHighlights.

For tips on avoiding problems with gym memberships, see Document 7.5.HealthSpa.

For tips on avoiding problems when buying exercise equipment, see Document 7.6.Equipment.

activity, specific activities, and real-life examples of how to meet the guidelines. As always, check with your health care provider before beginning an exercise program.

45. How can I gauge the intensity of an activity?

There are two ways to measure how intense an activity is: absolute intensity or relative intensity.

Absolute intensity is the amount of energy you use per minute of activity compared to when you're at rest. Absolute intensity is measured as **metabolic equivalent of task (MET)** intensity levels, which are expressed as multiples of RMR (resting metabolic rate—see Question 27). The rate of energy expenditure while you're at rest is one MET.

NOTE

At one MET the body's oxygen uptake is 3.5 milliliters per kilogram of body weight per minute for adults.

ON THE WEB

For a database of the MET values for different physical activities based on adult energy expenditure, visit:

https://sites.google.com/site/compendiumofphysicalactivities/Activity-Categories

For a list of MET values showing youth energy expenditure for different physical activities,[29] visit:

http://www.ijbnpa.org/content/supplementary/1479-5868-5-45-s1.pdf

- Light-intensity activities expend 1.1–2.9 times the energy expended at rest.

- Moderate-intensity activities expend 3.0–5.9 times the energy expended at rest.

- Vigorous-intensity activities expend 6.0 times or more the energy expended at rest.

Energy expenditure per unit body weight is higher in children, so the specific MET factor for an activity will differ for adults and children. Energy expenditure per unit body weight decreases as children get older and is equivalent to adult values by the time they're about 18 years old.

Relative intensity is how much effort you as an individual need to use to perform an activity. Usually, people who are less fit must expend more effort than people who are more physically fit to perform the same activity. You can estimate relative intensity using a scale of 0–10, where sitting is 0 and the highest possible effort is 10. On this scale, moderate-intensity activities would be 5–6 and vigorous-level activities would be 7–8.

For an overview of what counts toward meeting the physical activity guidelines, visit:

ON THE WEB

http://walking.about.com/od/fitness/a/exercise2007.htm

For three ways to gauge the intensity of your aerobic exercise, visit:

http://www.sparkpeople.com/resource/fitness_articles.asp?id=1044

For a list of moderate- and vigorous-intensity level activities for adults, visit:

http://www.cdc.gov/nccdphp/dnpa/physical/pdf/PA_Intensity_table_2_1.pdf

For a list of moderate- and vigorous-intensity level activities for children and adolescents, visit:

http://www.cdc.gov/physicalactivity/everyone/guidelines/what_counts.html

For a calorie calculator that provides results for more than 600 activities, visit:

TOOLS

http://www.webmd.com/diet/healthtool-fitness-calorie-counter

- Light-intensity activities are day-to-day (routine) activities that don't require much effort.

- Moderate-intensity activities are those that cause noticeable increases in breathing and heart rate. People doing this level of intensity can talk but can't sing.

- Vigorous-intensity activities are those that make your heart, lungs, and muscles work hard. People doing this level of activity can't say more than a few words without pausing for breath.

46. How many calories do different activities burn?

The number of calories you burn when you're engaged in a particular activity basically depends on three things: the level of intensity, your body composition (fat vs. lean), and the length of time you spend doing it. As we mentioned in Question 44, if you're younger than 18, your age matters too. Usually calorie calculators and tables that show calories expended for different activities use weight as a proxy for body composition. As a comparison, a 125-pound adult burns about 90 calories playing Frisbee for 30 minutes, while a 155-pound adult would burn about

112 calories and a 185-pound adult would burn about 133 calories in the same amount of time.[30]

47. Will exercise make me want to eat more?

Current research into the brain's food-reward systems has yielded mixed results as to whether exercise makes people want to eat more, but it does seem that some people, at least, can expect to feel more hungry after exercising. Here's a sampling of recent study results:

Two studies—one published in 2011, the other in 2012—seem to indicate that those who are physically fit to begin with may have less interest in eating after exercise, while those who are overweight and relatively sedentary may want to eat more after exercise.

To read more about these studies, visit:

http://well.blogs.nytimes.com/2012/04/16/does-exercise-make-you-overeat/

In contrast, another study published in 2012 found that all its participants responded less to food images after exercise, and that they didn't compensate for the exercise by eating more later.

To read more about this study, visit:

http://www.dailymail.co.uk/health/article-2202550/Work-appetite-Brisk-exercise-actually-REDUCES-hunger-pangs-scientists-claim.html

Meanwhile, research published in 2010 showed that exercise made rats' brains more responsive to insulin and leptin, which both have a role in regulating appetite.

To read more about this study, visit:

http://www.cbass.com/ExerciseCurbsAppetite.htm

The bottom line is that if you're hungry, you should eat something after a workout. Eating after exercising is fine and can help your body recover as long as you figure your snack into your total calorie budget for the day. The best post-workout snacks consist of about 60 percent carbohydrates (to replace glycogen, or muscle fuel), 25 percent protein (to help repair muscle tissue), and 15 percent fat. Examples include a slice of bread with peanut butter, yogurt with fruit, and dried fruit and nuts. You should also drink 16–20 ounces of water after your workout to replace fluid lost during exercise.

For more on post-workout snacking, visit:

http://www.sparkpeople.com/resource/nutrition_articles.asp?id=1082

48. Should I eat before exercising?

Glucose is a blood sugar that is the major source of energy for the body's cells; it comes primarily from the food we eat. Glycogen is the principle form in which glucose is stored in the body's tissues (particularly muscle and liver tissues).

For more on pre-workout eating, visit:

http://www.sparkpeople.com/resource/nutrition_articles.asp?id=1074

and

http://well.blogs.nytimes.com/2009/07/02/eating-to-fuel-exercise/

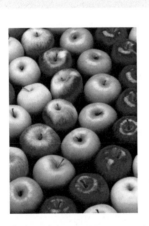

First, know that the fuel for your workout doesn't come from what you eat immediately before exercising, but rather from glycogen stores. The body's supply of glycogen should be enough for 3–4 hours of moderate-intensity exercise or 1–2 hours of vigorous-intensity exercise, more than sufficient for most workouts.

Blood sugar levels do drop after about 15 minutes of exercise, so eating before your workout can help if you tend to feel tired or weak during exercise. Experts recommend eating either a light snack (such as fruit) that's high in carbohydrates (which the body digests quickly) 30 minutes before you exercise, or a larger meal that's 50–60 percent carbohydrates (such as a peanut butter sandwich) an hour or two before your workout. It's important not to be too full during a workout, which can cause stomach discomfort or nausea, and you should avoid foods high in fat or fiber, which take a long time to digest.

People who aren't sensitive to their blood sugar levels dropping may not need to eat before moderate-intensity exercise, but probably will before a vigorous-intensity workout. Also, drinking 16–20 ounces of water before you exercise will make your workout more effective.

49. How can I fit exercise into my busy schedule?

Carving out time for exercise is probably the number one challenge for anyone who's trying to be more active. If you've been inactive for a while, a good first step is to look for opportunities to increase your activity level by making slight changes in your daily routine. For example, it's usually fairly easy to incorporate more walking into your day: parking

For other ways to incorporate more steps into your day, visit:

http://www.the-fitness-walking-guide.com/add-more-steps.html

as far as possible from the store when you go shopping, taking the stairs instead of the elevator, and using the restroom farthest away from your desk are all recommendations that have become clichés, but they really will help you increase your activity level without a big time commitment.

Also, keep in mind that household chores can count toward meeting the federal physical activity guidelines (some of these are listed on the list of moderate- and vigorous-intensity activities for adults in Question 45 On the Web). Washing windows, raking and bagging leaves, and digging in the garden are all moderate-intensity activities, and the last two will help you meet your strength-training goals as well. You can also crank up the cardio intensity of easier chores like vacuuming or folding laundry by setting time limits to complete them, or by incorporating extra moves for strength-training benefits.

ON THE WEB

For a list that compares the number of calories burned doing everyday household tasks to exercises like bicycling and ice-skating, visit:

http://www.dailymail.co.uk/health/article-93697/How-household-chores-shape.html

For tips on turning your chores into workouts, visit:

http://www.sharecare.com/question/good-workout-doing-household-chores

Now take a look at what you're already doing and what you need to add to meet the guidelines. Don't forget you're working toward substituting new (active) habits for old (inactive) habits, so start small and give yourself a chance to practice new routines before adding another goal (see Question 26). Here's how Jean, an inactive middle-aged woman profiled on pages 26–27 of the *Physical Guidelines for Americans*, built up her activity.

Her goals

Jean sets a goal of doing one hour a day of moderate-intensity aerobic activity five days a week (a total of 300 minutes a week). Weighing 220 pounds, Jean is obese and wants to lose about one pound of weight each week.

Starting out

Jean cuts back on her caloric intake and starts walking five minutes in the morning and five minutes in the evening most days of the week. She walks at a 2.5 mile-an-hour pace. Although physical activity tables show this to be light-intensity activity, for her level of fitness and fatness, it is appropriate moderate-intensity activity.

For tips on starting a walking program, see Document 7.7.Walking.

ON THE DVD

For sample activity routines, see Document 7.8.PARoutine.

For advice from eight experts on how to fit exercise into your schedule, visit:

ON THE WEB

http://www.sharecare.com/question/get-enough-exercise-with-busy-schedule

For more advice, visit:

http://exercise.about.com/od/fittinginexercise/a/busy_exercise.htm

and

http://www.everydayhealth.com/fitness/motivation/tips/being-active.aspx

To see how real people have made exercise a part of their lives, visit:

http://www.cdc.gov/physicalactivity/everyone/success/index.html

Two months later, Jean is comfortably walking 30 to 40 minutes at moderate intensity to and from her bus stop every day. She then adds variety to her activity by alternating among walking, riding a stationary cycle, and low-impact aerobics. She also begins muscle-strengthening activities, using elastic bands twice each week.

Scheduling exercise and making it a priority are both extremely important to a successful physical fitness program. If a conflict arises, it's fine to reschedule whatever activity you'd planned—as long as you treat the appointment as you would any other important commitment and keep it. Breaking activity into shorter sessions also will help you carve out time throughout the day.

50. How can I overcome other barriers to exercise?

Lack of time may be the biggest obstacle to increasing physical activity for most people, but there are others as well. Here are three common barriers and what you can do to get around them.

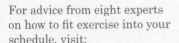

I'm too tired

Planning short exercise sessions—aerobic workouts can be as short as 10 minutes—not only helps you find time to exercise, it will also help you do a little even when you're tired. Often starting is the hardest part and you may find yourself exceeding your initial commitment once you get going. Scheduling activity throughout the day, and for times that you won't be as tired, will also help.

For other ways to push through fatigue, visit:

ON THE WEB

http://www.fitsugar.com/Favorite-Excuse-Working-Out-Im-Too-Tired-After-Work-155038

I'm embarrassed about my size

Even individuals who aren't overweight can feel self-conscious at the gym, particularly if they're new members—and certainly at facilities that attract people who like to show off. Exercising with workout videos at home, yard work or housework, and walking throughout the day can help you avoid joining a health club.

For tips on meeting the exercise challenges facing larger people, see Document 7.9.PASize.

If you feel awkward walking in public or do decide that a gym is the best alternative for you, teaming up with a friend can provide a lot of moral support. Just make sure that you check out the facility before you join to confirm that you'll feel comfortable.

For tips on choosing the gym that's right for you, visit:

http://www.msnbc.msn.com/id/15598063/ns/health-fitness/t/another-hurdle-exercise-embarrassment/#.UPf7xo4Tsb0

I can't afford to join a gym

Some of the same strategies that help you get around other obstacles to exercise will help if you can't afford a health club membership. Yard work, housework, and walking are all activities that won't cost you anything and will help you get in shape. You can also borrow exercise videos from the library or stream them for free if you have Internet access, and you can use household items such as gallons of water and canned goods as improvised dumbbells or other strength-training equipment.

For more ways to be active without spending a lot of money, visit:

http://nomoreplussize.com/2010/whats-your-excuse-i-cant-afford-a-gym/

For 10 ways to save money if you do join a gym, visit:

http://www.sparkpeople.com/resource/fitness_articles.asp?id=1258

There are many other reasons people give for avoiding exercise: some are afraid they'll hurt themselves, others think they aren't athletic enough, and still others think it has to be boring. But whatever hurdle seems to be standing in your way, there's usually at least one way around it. You just need to figure it out.

To conquer other barriers to exercise, see Document 7.10.Barriers.

51. How can I help my children to be more active?

To see how real moms have their kids help around the house, visit:

http://www.circleofmoms.com/stay-at-home-moms/children-cleaning-up-help-with-housework-528517#_

ON THE WEB

For advice on getting your children to be more active, visit:

http://www.healthychildren.org/English/healthy-living/fitness/pages/Encouraging-Your-Child-to-be-Physically-Active.aspx?nfstatus=401&nftoken=00000000-0000-0000-0000-000000000000&nfstatusdescription=ERROR%3a+No+local+token

ON THE WEB

For ways to make exercise fun for kids in grade school, visit:

http://www.circleofmoms.com/article/5-ways-make-exercise-fun-gradeschoolers-05777

For information on the nonphysical benefits of play, visit:

http://greatergood.berkeley.edu/gg_live/parenting_videos/video/positive_parenting_get_out_and_play/

For tips to help you talk to your teen about becoming more active, visit:

http://www.pamf.org/teen/parents/health/exercise.html

For five ways to help an inactive teen get more exercise, visit:

http://www.webmd.com/parenting/raising-fit-kids/move/get-teens-moving?page=1

To learn more about how different kinds of screen time affect kids, visit:

http://greatergood.berkeley.edu/gg_live/parenting_videos/video/positiive_parenting_screentime/

ON THE WEB

Parents who are active are great role models for their children, and the suggestions outlined in Questions 49 and 50 can help both you and your children get more exercise. Expecting your kids to help with household chores and yard work is normal, so don't hesitate to give them age-appropriate assignments from an early age—even if they don't complete their tasks perfectly, involving them will help keep them active, teach them responsibility, and let them know that helping out is part of being a family.

As we mentioned in Question 42, physical activity is essential for children: to help them maintain a healthy weight, to reduce the need for calorie cutting when they do need to lose weight, and to set the stage for a lifetime of being physically active. Children should be encouraged to be active from a young age and will be more likely to want to be if activities are fun and varied. Having company helps too—whether it's other children, a parent, or the whole family.

Screen time—TV, computer, video games, etc.—can be a big barrier to children and adolescents getting enough exercise. In this, too, you need to be a good role model by showing your children that activities that get you up and moving can be just as much fun as watching TV or playing a video game. The American Academy of Pediatrics recommends a maximum of 1–2 hours of total screen time a day for children older than two and discourages screen time altogether for children under age two.

Screen time is not uniformly bad, but too much does interfere with other things that children and adolescents need for their mental and physical development. There's also lots of research linking too much television viewing to childhood (and adult!) obesity. Experts speculate that excessive TV viewing may promote obesity by taking up time that otherwise might be spent being active, by encouraging poor eating habits through advertising, by providing more opportunities for unhealthy snacking, and even by interfering with sleep.[31] One study found that youth who watched more than five hours of TV a day were almost five times as likely to be overweight as those who watched two hours or less.[32]

Planning activities that the family can do together shows your children that getting exercise is normal and part of enjoying life. Riding bikes together, walking after dinner, and flying kites at the park are all low-cost activities that will help everyone in the family get more exercise and bring you together. When paired with sensible eating habits, time spent being active as a family will help your children develop healthy habits that last a lifetime.

 For tips on limiting screen time for your children, visit:

http://www.healthychildren.org/english/family-life/media/pages/The-Benefits-of-Limiting-TV.aspx

and

http://www.kidseatgreat.com/setting-media-limits.htm

 For advice on helping your child eat healthy and be physically active, see Document 7.11.HelpChild.

For five steps to creating a healthy home, see Document 7.12.TakeAction.

To help teenagers take charge of their health, see Document 7.13.Teen.

To see how parents can help their children become more active, see Document 7.14.PAParents.

For ways the family can be active together, see Document 7.15.PAFamily.

For a calendar to track healthy eating and physical activity for the family, see Document 7.16.FamCalendar.

For a log to track family screen time, see Document 7.17.FamScreen.

For a chart to track family health goals, see Document 7.18.FamGoal.

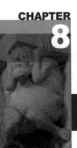 8 *Drug Treatments for Obesity*

52. When should drug treatments for obesity be considered?

No drug can cure obesity, and medication should be used only to support combined therapy (low-calorie diet, physical activity, behavior therapy) in certain patients after six months of combined therapy. Your doctor may recommend drug treatment if:

- Your body mass index (BMI) is 30 or greater

For an overview of some of the medications used to treat obesity in the United States, see Document 8.1.ObesMeds.
ON THE DVD

- Your BMI is greater than 27 and you also have medical complications of obesity, such as diabetes, high blood pressure, or sleep apnea

53. What drug treatments are available to treat obesity?

Medications currently used for weight loss work either by suppressing appetite, altering metabolism, or inhibiting calorie absorption. Several of the drugs most commonly prescribed follow; some have been approved by the FDA to treat obesity, while others are prescribed off label. **Off-label use** is the practice of prescribing medication for conditions or time periods that have not been approved by the FDA.

Phentermine

Phentermine is an anorectic drug, or one that works by suppressing appetite. It was approved by the FDA in 1959 for adults and is marketed under a number of brand names, including Teva Pharmaceuticals' **Adipex-P®** and Medeva Pharmaceuticals' **Ionamin®**, and as a generic. It is typically prescribed only for short-term use since it can be habit forming.

Side effects of phentermine can include:

- Dry mouth
- Unpleasant taste
- Diarrhea
- Constipation
- Vomiting

Serious side effects can include:

- Increased blood pressure
- Heart palpitations
- Restlessness
- Dizziness

Diethylpropion

Diethylpropion is a **stimulant** (a drug that temporarily improves mental or physical functioning) prescribed as an appetite suppressant. Diethylpropion hydrochloride is marketed under several brand names, including **Tenuate®** and **Tenuate Dospan®** (both from Merrell Pharmaceuticals), and was first approved by the FDA for adult use in 1959. It can be habit forming and is recommended only for short-term use. Diethylpropion is not recommended for individuals with pulmonary hypertension, severe coronary artery disease, glaucoma, overactive thyroid, or severe or uncontrolled high blood pressure.

Side effects can include:

- Dry mouth
- Unpleasant taste
- Restlessness
- Anxiety
- Dizziness
- Depression

Serious side effects can include:

- Fast or irregular heartbeat
- Heart palpitations
- Blurred vision
- Skin rash
- Itching
- Difficulty breathing

ON THE WEB

For more information about phentermine, visit:

http://www.nlm.nih.gov/medlineplus/druginfo/meds/a682187.html

For more information about diethylpropion, visit:

http://www.nlm.nih.gov/medlineplus/druginfo/meds/a682037.html

Topiramate

Topiramate is a prescription **anticonvulsant** medication used to control seizures in children and adults with epilepsy, and children with Lennox-Gastaut syndrome. Available from Janssen Pharmaceuticals under the brand name **Topamax®**, it is also frequently prescribed to prevent migraine headaches.

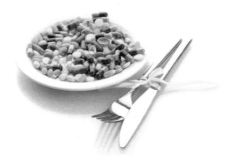

The FDA has not approved topiramate as a weight loss medication, but because weight loss is a side effect some doctors have prescribed it off label for this purpose. Women who are pregnant or planning to become pregnant should be aware that infants born to women taking topiramate are at increased risk for birth defects, specifically cleft lip and cleft palate (a gap in the lip or palate, respectively).

Side effects of topiramate can include:

- Numbness and tingling
- Upper respiratory tract infections
- Depression or suicidal thoughts
- Speech and memory problems

Serious side effects can include:

- Eye pain or blurred vision
- Slow, irregular, or pounding heartbeat
- Trouble breathing

Phentermine-topiramate

Phentermine-topiramate is a combination prescription drug being marketed under the name **Qsymia™**. After voting against approval in 2010, the FDA approved Qsymia for adult use in 2012 following VIVUS's release of additional results from clinical trials and a plan that limits distribution to certified mail-order pharmacies. It contains phentermine, an appetite suppressant, and topiramate, an anticonvulsant (see previous sections on phentermine and topiramate).

Qsymia can cause birth defects, so women of childbearing age should take it only if they are using effective birth control and their pregnancy tests are negative before and while using it. It should not be used in patients with glaucoma or hyperthyroidism, and is not recommended for individuals who have experienced unstable heart disease or stroke within the last six months. If patients fail to lose 3 percent of their weight within 12 weeks doctors may either increase the dosage or stop treatment.

Side effects of phentermine-topiramate can include:

* Increased heart rate
* Tingling of hands and feet
* Altered taste sensation
* Insomnia
* Dizziness
* Dry mouth
* Constipation

Serious side effects can include:

* Suicidal thoughts
* Memory or comprehension problems
* Sleep disorders
* Vision changes

For more information about topiramate, visit:

http://www.nlm.nih.gov/
medlineplus/druginfo/meds/
a697012.html#other-uses

For the FDA's announcement approving Qsymia, visit:

http://www.fda.gov/NewsEvents/Newsroom/
PressAnnouncements/ucm312468.htm

Orlistat

Orlistat is marketed by Hoffman-LaRoche as the prescription drug **Xenical®** in most countries, and as the over-the-counter (OTC) drug **Allī®** in the United States and the United Kingdom. It is a **lipase inhibitor**, which means that it works by preventing some fat from being absorbed in the stomach and intestines. Fat that is not absorbed is eliminated in the stool. The Food and Drug Administration (FDA) has approved it for use in adults and in children age 12 and up. The agency approved Xenical in 1999 and Allī in 2007.

For more information about orlistat, visit:

http://www.nlm.nih.gov/
medlineplus/druginfo/meds/
a601244.html

For the FDA's 2009 announcement relabeling orlistat to include information about liver injury, visit:

http://www.fda.gov/Drugs/DrugSafety/
PostmarketDrugSafetyInformation
forPatientsandProviders/
ucm213040.htm

Side effects of orlistat can include:

* Changes in bowel movements, including oily and loose stools and frequency and urgency in elimination
* Gas
* Stomach cramps

Severe liver injury is a potentially serious, if rare, risk of using orlistat. Signs of liver injury can include:

- Itching
- Yellow eyes or skin
- Dark urine
- Light-colored stools
- Loss of appetite

Lorcaserin

After initially voting against approval in 2010, an FDA panel approved prescription drug **Belviq®** (lorcaserin hydrochloride) for use in adults in 2012, after a new round of studies by Arena Pharmaceuticals. **Lorcaserin** works by activating the serotonin 2C receptor (which influences appetite) in the brain. Activating this receptor may help people feel full even after eating less. The FDA recommends that the drug be discontinued if patients fail to lose 5 percent of their body weight after 12 weeks, as continued treatment is unlikely to be successful for those individuals.

Because weight loss offers no benefit in pregnancy and may harm the fetus, pregnant women shouldn't take Lorcaserin. The FDA recommends that lorcaserin be used with caution in patients with congestive heart failure, because the number of serotonin 2B receptors (which are thought to have a role in damaging heart valves) may be increased in people with this condition, and has required that the manufacturer conduct studies to assess cardiovascular risks from the drug.

For nondiabetic patients, side effects can include:

- Headache
- Dizziness
- Fatigue
- Nausea
- Dry mouth
- Constipation

In diabetic patients, side effects can include:

- Low blood sugar (hypoglycemia)
- Headache
- Back pain
- Cough
- Fatigue

For the FDA's announcement approving Belviq, visit:

http://www.fda.gov/NewsEvents/ Newsroom/PressAnnouncements/ ucm309993.htm

ON THE WEB

Rare but serious side effects can include:

* A chemical imbalance (serotonin syndrome)
* Suicidal thoughts
* Psychiatric problems
* Problems with memory or comprehension

Bupropion

Bupropion is a prescription antidepressant marketed under the brand names **Wellbutrin®** (Valeant Pharmaceuticals) and **Zyban®** (GlaxoSmithKline), among others. Bupropion is not recommended for children younger than age 18, although doctors may decide that it's the best course of treatment for some individuals. The drug was originally introduced in the United States in 1984 to treat depression but was pulled from the market due to a high incidence of seizures. Bupropion was reintroduced in 1989 and approved by the FDA for smoking cessation in 1997. Patients taking bupropion have experienced weight loss as a side effect, leading to its off-label use in weight loss treatment programs.

Side effects of bupropion can include:

* Drowsiness
* Excitement
* Dry mouth
* Dizziness
* Headache
* Nausea

Serious side effects can include:

* Seizures
* Confusion
* Hallucinations
* Difficulty breathing or swallowing
* Chest pain
* Muscle or joint pain

ON THE WEB

For more information about bupropion, visit:

http://www.nlm.nih.gov/medlineplus/druginfo/meds/a695033.html

54. What about herbal supplements?

The FDA regulates dietary supplements as foods, not drugs. Supplements therefore are not subjected to the same safety and efficacy testing as drugs and do not undergo an approval process. The FDA also monitors product information (labeling, claims, etc.) and is

For more about dietary supplements and how they're regulated, see Document 8.2.DietSupp.

For tips on making informed decisions about supplements, visit:

http://www.fda.gov/food/dietarysupplements/consumerinformation/ucm110567.htm

For tips directed at older supplement users, visit:

http://www.fda.gov/Food/DietarySupplements/ConsumerInformation/ucm110493.htm

To check the FDA Web site for supplement alerts, visit:

http://www.fda.gov/Food/DietarySupplements/Alerts/default.htm

For additional information about supplements and links to other resources, check out the Web site for the NIH's Office of Dietary Supplements (ODS):

http://ods.od.nih.gov/

To test your supplement savvy, see Document 8.3.SuppSavvy.

responsible for taking action against unsafe supplements once they've reached the market. The Federal Trade Commission (FTC) regulates advertising for dietary supplements and investigates complaints about false or misleading health claims posted on the Internet.

Given that dietary supplements aren't tested for safety or effectiveness, you should be extremely cautious about claims made about them and any hidden health risks. It's a good idea to check with your health care provider and check the FDA Web site for alerts before taking any supplement.

The marketing terms used to promote supplements, along with the fact that they are widely available, may suggest to consumers that supplements are a healthful and natural way to lose weight. Again, checking with your doctor or pharmacist can help you use supplements safely.

There are a huge number of supplements marketed as weight loss aids, and not much in the way of proof that any of them work. Here's a sampling of some of these supplements.

Acai berry

Acai (pronounced ah-sigh-EE)—also known as the Amazonian palm berry—comes from a palm tree native to Central and South America. Products are available as juices, powders, tablets, and capsules. No independent studies substantiate weight loss claims.

Bitter orange

Bitter orange, or *zhi shi*, comes from a tree of the same name native to parts of Asia and Africa that is now grown in California and Florida, and throughout the Mediterranean region. Many herbal weight loss products have replaced **ephedra**, which was banned by the FDA in 2004, with concentrated extracts of bitter orange peel. There is insufficient evidence to support the use of bitter orange in a weight loss program.

For more on acai, see Document 8.4.Acai.

For more on bitter orange, see Document 8.5.BitOrange.

Chromium

Trivalent chromium, or **chromium 3+**, exists in trace amounts in certain foods (meats, whole-grain products, and some fruits, vegetables, and herbs).[33] It helps insulin to metabolize carbohydrates, fat, and protein, but more research is needed to establish the nature of its roles in the body. Studies done to date have not supported claims that chromium supplements help to reduce body fat and increase lean muscle.

For more on chromium, see Document 8.6.Chromium.

Green coffee bean extract

The active ingredient in **green coffee bean extract**, which is derived from unroasted coffee beans, is **chlorogenic acid**. The compound is said to decrease the rate at which sugar is released into the body and cue the body to burn glucose and fat. Chlorogenic acid isn't present in the beans that we use to brew coffee because the roasting process removes it. A 2012 study that tested its weight loss properties showed "statistically significant reductions in weight, BMI, [and] percent body fat" without dietary or lifestyle changes.[34] Additional research is needed to confirm green coffee bean extract's effectiveness as a weight loss supplement.

To view a segment from the *Dr. Oz Show* on green coffee bean extract, visit:

http://www.youtube.com/watch?v=kNXRiBBKk78

Green tea

Green tea is produced by steaming fresh leaves of the *Camellia sinensis* plant. The leaves can be brewed and consumed as a beverage, or processed to produce capsules made from extracts. There is not yet reliable data to prove green tea's usefulness as a weight loss aid.

For more on green tea, see Document 8.7.GreenTea.

Guar gum

Guar gum is produced from the seeds of the guar bean, which is native to India. It is used by the food industry in a variety of applications, including as a thickener for dairy products, as a binder for meat, and as an additive in many foods to extend shelf life. As a dietary fiber it helps to promote a feeling of fullness after eating, and it was promoted widely in a number of weight loss products in the 1980s. Reports of esophageal blockage, hospitalizations, and one death caused the FDA to ban its use in OTC weight loss aids. Nevertheless, it is still sold online (and perhaps elsewhere) as a weight loss aid.

Hoodia

Hoodia, or Kalahari cactus, is a succulent plant native to the Kalahari Desert. Native African Bushmen have long used hoodia stems as an appetite suppressant. Stems and roots can be dried to make extracts—which are then made into chewable tablets, capsules, and powders—or processed into liquid extracts and teas. Hoodia products frequently include other ingredients, such as green tea or chromium picolinate.[35] No studies have been published about use of hoodia in humans.

For more on hoodia, see Document 8.8.Hoodia.

ON THE DVD

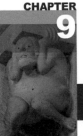

CHAPTER 9 *Surgical Treatments for Obesity*

55. When should surgical treatments for obesity be considered?

Bariatric surgery (weight loss surgery) is usually a last resort for individuals who haven't been able to lose sufficient weight through changes in diet and exercise—possibly supported by medication—alone. Patients who undergo surgery still must commit to a healthful diet, portion control, and increased exercise or they can gain lost weight back. The FDA has only approved bariatric surgery for people who are age 18 and older, but the creator of the Lap-Band® gastric banding system is currently seeking approval to make the system available to those age 14 and up (see the section on adjustable gastric banding later in this chapter for a description of this technology).

Doctors generally consider surgery only for adult patients who have:

- A body mass index (BMI) of 40 or greater
- A BMI greater than 35 with an obesity-related medical condition, such as diabetes, high blood pressure, or severe sleep apnea

and young adults who have:

- A BMI of 40 or greater
- Reached their adult height
- Obesity-related health problems

The term bariatric surgery comes from the Greek words *baros* (weight) and *iatrikos* (medicine).

People must typically meet other medical guidelines to qualify for bariatric surgery, so patient characteristics other than BMI usually are taken into consideration as well, including:

- Experiences with weight loss, diet and exercise habits
- Medical factors impacting surgical risk
- Mental health
- Motivation to maintain post-surgery lifestyle changes
- Age

For more on pre-surgery evaluation, visit:

http://www.mayoclinic.com/print/gastric-bypass-surgery/WT00031/METHOD=print

56. What kinds of surgical treatments are available to treat obesity?

Bariatric surgery can be restrictive (meaning it works by limiting the intake of food and liquids by reducing the size of the stomach), malabsorptive (in which part of the digestive tract is bypassed, decreasing the absorption of calories and nutrients in the small intestine), or a combination of the two.

Surgery is performed using either the open method, which requires an 8–10 inch abdominal incision, or the laparoscopic method, in which several small keyhole incisions are made in the abdomen to allow for the passage of surgical tools and a laparoscope (which projects images of the surgery on a computer monitor). The most common types of bariatric surgery performed in the United States are adjustable gastric banding (also known as lap banding), Roux-en-Y gastric bypass surgery, vertical sleeve gastrectomy (or gastric sleeve), and biliopancreatic diversion with a duodenal switch (or simply duodenal switch).

Adjustable gastric banding

Adjustable gastric banding (AGB), or lap banding, is a restrictive procedure. It was originally approved in the United States for patients age 18 and older who meet the criteria described in Question 55, but in February 2011 the FDA expanded approval to include patients with a BMI of 30 or greater with at least one obesity-related medical condition. Lap banding is the least invasive type of bariatric surgery and is also completely reversible. As it becomes more popular it's beginning to replace vertical banded gastroplasty (VGB), or stomach stapling, which is considered "severely dangerous" by the American Medical Association.

▼ FIGURE 9.1
Adjustable gastric band (lap band).

Adjustable Gastric Band (Lap Band)

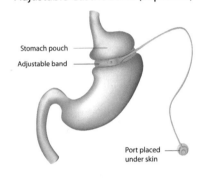

Stomach pouch
Adjustable band
Port placed
under skin

SOURCE: Diagram by Alila Sao Mai.

During AGB, a silicone band lined with an inflatable balloon is placed around the top of the stomach, creating a smaller pouch and restricting food consumption (see Figure 9.1). A port placed beneath the skin allows the inflation of the band to be adjusted after surgery to meet patient needs.

Roux-en-Y gastric bypass

Roux-en-Y gastric bypass (RYGB) surgery is both a restrictive and malabsorptive procedure, because it limits food intake and reduces calorie absorption. It is one variant of gastric bypass surgery (bypasses differ in how the small intestine is reattached). All gastric bypass procedures divide the stomach into a small upper pouch that serves as the new stomach, and a lower pouch that doesn't receive food but still secretes gastric juices. Once a smaller stomach is created, a piece of the small intestine is cut. One end is connected to the new stomach and the other end is attached lower down on the small intestine so that digestion bypasses the lower compartment (see Figure 9.2). Gastric bypass is

▼ FIGURE 9.2
Roux-en-Y gastric bypass.

Roux-en-Y Gastric Bypass (RNY)

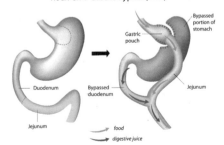

Gastric
pouch
Bypassed
portion of
stomach
Duodenum
Bypassed
duodenum
Jejunum
Jejunum
food
digestive juice

SOURCE: Diagram by Alila Sao Mai.

the most common form of bariatric surgery performed in the United States because it usually results in greater weight loss than other procedures while presenting reasonable risks and limited side effects.

Vertical sleeve gastrectomy

Vertical sleeve gastrectomy (VSG), or **gastric sleeve**, is a restrictive procedure that removes about 75 percent of the stomach (the appendix and gall bladder are also removed). The remaining stomach resembles a curved tube or sleeve (see Figure 9.3). VSG does not reroute the small intestine.

ON THE WEB

For a video of how VSG reconfigures the stomach, visit:

http://www.youtube.com/watch?v=bEZu93jiPmc

VSG is normally used with patients whose medical issues and/or high body weight increases the risk of other bariatric procedures. Previously it served as the first step in the two-step biliopancreatic-diversion-with-duodenal-switch procedure discussed next, but doctors have found that some patients have been able to lose sufficient weight with VSG alone. Researchers have not yet determined the number of people who will eventually need the second part of the surgery.

▼ FIGURE 9.3
Vertical sleeve gastrectomy.

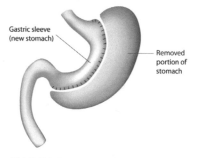

SOURCE: Diagram by Alila Sao Mai.

Biliopancreatic diversion with a duodenal switch

The **biliopancreatic diversion with a duodenal switch (BPD-DS)**, or **duodenal switch (DS)**, has both restrictive and malabsorptive features. It is a complex, two-part surgery that's usually reserved for patients with a BMI of at least 50 due to its risks. BPD-DS should be distinguished from the procedure called **biliopancreatic diversion (BPD)**, which removes a different section of the stomach as well as the **pyloric valve** (the ring of muscle that controls the passage of food from the stomach to the duodenum).

The first step in BPD-DS involves removing about 75 percent of the stomach through a vertical sleeve gastrectomy (see previous description and Figure 9.3).

For a before-and-after illustration of how BPD-DS changes the configuration of the digestive system, visit:

http://www.kettering-sycamorewls.org/swfs/BPD.swf

For a look at how AGB, VGB, RYGB, and BPD are performed, visit:

http://www.youtube.com/watch?v=I8D8zpLqpw8

For guidance on who makes a good candidate for bariatric surgery, information on cost and risks, and an overview of the bariatric procedures discussed here, see Document 9.1.ObesSurg.

For links to additional resources on bariatric surgery, including post-surgery nutritional information and current research and clinical trials, visit:

http://www.nlm.nih.gov/medlineplus/weightlosssurgery.html#cat1

During the second step a large portion of the small intestine is rerouted to form one common channel and two separate ones. The shorter of the separate channels (called the **digestive loop**) carries food from the new stomach to the common channel, while the longer channel (the **biliopancreatic loop**) carries bile from the liver to the common channel.

After surgery, food bypasses most of the duodenum (the first section of the small intestine), making the distance between the stomach and the colon much shorter and limiting the amount of calories that are absorbed. Redirecting bile from the liver also reduces the body's absorption of calories and fat. These malabsorptive effects, combined with the restrictive effect of reducing stomach size, results in the loss of a high percentage of excess weight.

People who are considering bariatric surgery should remember that all surgery carries risks and that certain procedures may not be appropriate for everyone. They should also keep in mind that bariatric surgery is expensive and that insurance coverage varies.

Given the scale of the obesity problem worldwide, bariatric surgery will continue to be an important option for people who are unable to sustain weight loss through other methods.

Weight Plateaus and Weight Maintenance

CHAPTER 10

57. What do I need to know about weight loss plateaus?

Weight loss plateaus are those all-but-inevitable periods when the scale doesn't move, even though you're being careful to follow your weight loss program. A plateau is a transitional period during which your metabolism adjusts to your body's new, lower weight. Depending on how much weight you have to lose, you should expect to experience more than one plateau before you reach your goal weight, and as you get closer to that weight you may find it harder to break through plateaus.

One explanation for plateaus is **set-point theory**, which was developed in 1982 to explain the common difficulty of long-term weight loss maintenance. The theory argues that genetics programs the body to maintain weight and fat at a certain level (or within a certain range), and that consequently as you lose weight and fat the body adjusts metabolism to return to its natural set point.

Research showing that obese individuals have metabolisms similar to those of individuals who have never been overweight has challenged set-point theory, but other studies have supported it, and recent reviews of bariatric surgery outcomes have suggested that surgery can help the body establish a new set point (although more investigation is needed).[36] Scientists continue to investigate whether the body does have a natural set point and, if so, whether it works in the manner proposed by the researchers who developed the theory, but for now the theory stands.

What we do know is that it takes fewer calories to fuel a smaller body (see Question 27), that the body continually adjusts metabolism in response to changes in either calorie intake or activity level (see Question 30), and that it's easier to gain weight than to lose it (see Question 42). These factors are sufficient in themselves to bring about weight plateaus.

Plateaus are typically defined as 3–4 weeks without weight loss, but their timing within the weight loss cycle seems to depend to some degree on the individual. If you stop losing

> **NOTE**
> Plateaus also occur with weight gain. When calories consumed are greater than calories burned, initially you'll gain weight, but then your metabolism will increase because of your extra body weight. When a balance is met, the weight gain will stop and your new weight will be maintained.

weight fewer than four weeks into a diet, however, in all likelihood you're not dealing with a weight loss plateau. Many would argue, in fact, that you're probably not experiencing a plateau unless you've been dieting for at least six months, while others say that plateaus naturally occur after you've lost about 10 percent of your body weight.

Regardless, before you assume that you've started to plateau, ask yourself the following questions:

- Are your goals realistic? Make sure you're not sending your body into starvation mode by eating too few calories (see Question 29), that you're not thinking you'll lose more weight each week than is reasonable, and that your end goal is realistic for your height and the effort you're willing to put in.

- Have you set a new calorie budget for your current weight? At a minimum, you should be reevaluating your calorie needs after every 10 pounds that you lose, but looking at your budget about every month or so is even better. We'll use Ted and Susan from Question 28 as an example: Ted is 6 feet 3 inches and weighs 230 pounds, Susan is 5 feet 5 inches and weighs 150 pounds, and both are 45 years old with a moderate level of activity.

  Using the calorie-calculator link in Question 28, we see that Ted needs 3125 calories a day to maintain his current weight. If he loses 10 pounds he'll need 70 fewer (3055 calories) to support his new weight of 220 pounds. Meanwhile, at 150 pounds Susan needs 2060 calories, and if she loses 10 pounds she'll also require 70 fewer calories (1990) to maintain her new weight of 140 pounds. But if each maintain their initial calorie budgets, they'd eat 25,550 more calories (70 × 365) than they need over the course of a year. Assuming 3500 calories per pound, that's the equivalent of about 7 pounds.

- Are you staying within your calorie budget? It takes a certain level of commitment to record what you're eating accurately and consistently, and it's not uncommon for dieters to become more lax about tracking as time goes on. Beverages (particularly alcohol and soda), sauces, salad dressings, condiments, and portion size are all likely culprits in calorie creep. Bad habits like finishing your child's meal and tasting too much when you're cooking can also contribute to overages. Make sure you're consuming what you think you are.

ON THE WEB

For more on how to tell if you're experiencing a plateau, visit:

http://www.psychologytoday.com/blog/the-instinct-diet/200903/plateaus-why-they-happen-and-how-get-through-them
and

http://www.huffingtonpost.com/2011/10/11/weight loss-plateau_n_1004197.html

• Are you getting enough physical activity? In Chapter 7, we talked about becoming more active gradually, and that's fine. At the same time, though, you need to work toward a certain level of physical activity—in ways big and small—in order to lose weight. Be easy enough on yourself to avoid injuries and to accommodate your schedule, but be hard enough on yourself to ask whether it's time to be doing a bit more.

If you've established that your goals, eating, and activity levels are all where they should be and that you're experiencing a plateau, you'll need to take action to push through it. We'll talk about what you can do next, but keep in mind that the most difficult part of a plateau can be maintaining resolve and not giving up . . . so if you need a reminder about changing old habits, review Chapter 5.

For more about weight loss plateaus, visit:

http://www.builtlean.com/2012/05/22/weight loss-plateau/

58. How can I overcome a weight loss plateau?

Overcoming a weight loss plateau basically requires shaking the body up by modifying your routine. Your aim is to make small changes in both your diet and your exercise regimen to dislodge your body from its holding pattern. The tactics that work for one individual may not work for another, so count on experimenting with a few different things to find what works for you. Trying one diet adjustment coupled with one activity adjustment at a time will help you identify what helped.

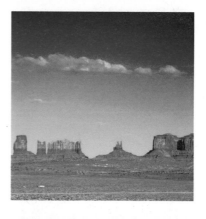

Diet

Experts often suggest that you try reducing calories consumed to break a plateau, starting with around 100 per day and gradually increasing the reduction to 200–300 per day as needed. Given the difficulties inherent in figuring out a calorie budget (particularly as your weight changes) it makes sense that decreasing your daily calories should be your first step, assuming you're not already at a minimum calorie level. Here are three other strategies that may help:

• Increase calories by 100 a day for a week or two. This seems counterintuitive, but as we discussed in Question 30 it becomes more difficult to lose fat as the body becomes leaner and wants to hold onto fat reserves. Temporarily eating more can help the body relax about losing fat. If you're increasing your physical activity at the same time, the extra calories will also provide fuel to build muscle. More muscle means a higher metabolism, which means more calories burned. You only want to increase calorie intake slightly and for a limited time.

- Eat more often. As discussed in Question 23, eating six small meals a day helps some people control hunger, food cravings, and blood sugar better than when they're eating three large meals. It can also help limit how many calories are stored as fat. Because insulin increases the storage of fat in fat cells and prevents fat cells from releasing fat for energy, and because your body releases less insulin in response to smaller meals than larger ones, more frequent meals keep insulin levels lower and more stable. The less insulin you have in your blood, the more fat you burn, and the less you store.

- Check your nutrient mix. In Chapter 6, we talked a lot about what healthy eating is and the importance of a balanced diet. As we know, the nutrients you get from a 100-calorie chocolate bar are quite different from the nutrients you get from a 100-calorie apple. Healthy eating is important because it supports—well, your health. And good health supports your body's systems working as they should and having the energy and stamina to carry on with a good level of physical activity.

If you're staying within your calorie budget but are hungry all the time, try bumping up the fiber in your diet so that you'll feel more full. Also, look at what you've been eating to make sure you're not overdoing the fat and empty calories. Research has yielded mixed results on whether changing the proportion of carbohydrates, protein, and fat really matters in weight loss, but some people say that changing up the mix slightly—particularly bumping up protein levels—has helped them end weight plateaus. Also, keep in mind that you need protein to build muscle.

If you're working with a health care professional, the possibility of food sensitivities and allergies, nutrient deficiencies, and hormonal imbalances will have been explored when you're developing your weight

To read how eating more can help you lose weight, visit:

 ON THE WEB

http://www.thepostgame.com/blog/training-table/201209/5-reasons-why-eating-more-helps-you-lose-weight-0

For more on how underlying medical problems can interfere with weight management, visit:

 ON THE WEB

http://mymix967.com/view/full_story/20656376/article-How-to-blast-through-your-weight-loss-plateau?instance=Fashion loss program. If you're really struggling with weight loss in general, or can't seem to break a stubborn weight plateau, though, you should consider being evaluated for undiagnosed medical problems.

Physical Activity

As time goes on your body becomes more efficient at performing the same activities, so you'll need to increase the intensity (and perhaps the frequency) of your routine and switch up individual components on a regular basis, especially if you've hit a weight loss plateau. Opinions vary on how often you should do this, but unless you're an athlete you shouldn't have to do it any more frequently than every 2–4 weeks (the body takes about two weeks to adapt to an exercise).

When the body becomes efficient at an exercise, you burn fewer calories and less fat, and build less muscle mass. Bumping up the intensity of cardio exercises improves your cardiovascular health at the same time that it keeps calories burned from dropping. Likewise, increasing the intensity of strength-training activities will prevent calories expended from decreasing as you build muscle—and more muscle means a higher BMR and more calories burned (see Question 27).

 ON THE WEB

For a look at how the body builds muscle and why you need a certain amount of calories to support the process, visit:

http://www.ehow.com/how-does_5143360_body-build-muscle.html

The changes you make to your routine need not be extreme, and probably shouldn't be, because completely changing your workout will make it harder to keep track of your baseline as you increase the intensity of an exercise. Switching out some exercises for others on a regular basis, however, will keep you from getting bored, ensure that you're working all muscle groups, and, as mentioned earlier, keep you burning enough fat and calories to lose weight and build muscle mass.

If you can afford it, a personal trainer can be very helpful not only in designing an exercise program specific to your needs but also in helping you to decide when and how to modify an existing program. Here are some general suggestions for shaking up your routine:

* Increase intensity either by increasing the force of an exercise or by doing it longer. For example, if you're walking five times a week for 30 minutes (an aerobic activity that also strengthens your muscles—see Question 43), you could either pick up your pace by a half-mile per hour or by walking for 15 minutes more.

* Increase frequency by adding daily or weekly workouts. For example, you could add a sixth day of walking to your routine

or try doing two walks a day. If you choose the latter and can't fit an hour in during the day, start with two 20-minute sessions (remember that aerobic activities shouldn't be shorter than 10 minutes).

- Substitute another activity on some days of the week. For instance, swim laps two days a week and walk the other three. If you are trying to get both cardio and strength-training benefits from the same exercise, make sure to consider whether the activity you substitute will provide the same benefits—you may want to bump up your strength-training regimen if it won't.

- Switch off every week between two programs. Building variety into your program from the beginning should extend the length of time before you need to incorporate new changes and provide the added bonus of keeping boredom at bay. During week one, for example, you would walk on Monday, Wednesday, and Friday and ride your bicycle on Tuesday and Thursday. During week two you'd cycle on Monday, Wednesday, and Friday and walk on Tuesday and Thursday.

These examples use the cardio part of your routine as illustrations, but you should change the strength-training part of your workout too. You can modify muscle-building activities by changing the order in which you do them, the number of repetitions and/or number of sets you do, how fast you do each repetition, and the length or number of rest periods you take in between sets or exercises. In fact, adding a couple of sessions of strength training to your regimen may be one of the better ways to break a weight loss plateau because of the muscle mass you'll build.

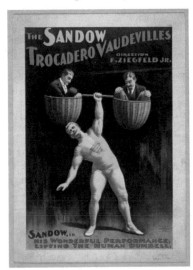

Many experts consider high intensity interval training (HIIT)—or simply interval training—as one of the most effective ways to overcome weight loss plateaus (and one of the most effective ways to exercise, period). Interval training alternates short high-intensity work periods with lower-intensity "rest" periods within one aerobic activity. It's said to burn fat and improve fitness more quickly than periods of constant, moderate-intensity cardio activity. If you have heart problems interval training will probably not be appropriate for you, and it's usually too intense for people who are just beginning an exercise program. As with any new exercise program, you should consult your health care provider before you begin.

For results of one study on the effectiveness of interval training, visit:

http://www.sciencedaily.com/releases/2007/06/070627140103.htm

For an overview of interval training that includes some sample workouts, visit:

http://www.winchestermed.com/articles/breaking-through-your-weight loss-plateau-with-interval-training/

For a video that helps beginners get started with interval training, visit:

http://www.youtube.com/watch?v=WRfx7A3LzzU

Attitude

There's another way to look at a plateau, and that's as an opportunity to rest for six months and build back any muscle that's been lost during the initial weight loss phase. If you're comfortable with this approach, chances are your body will break through the plateau naturally after this period is up. During the lull your mission would be to stick very closely to the calorie budget for your new weight and continue improving your physical activity levels. After six months you'd decrease calories again and start the next phase of weight loss.

For more on appreciating weight loss plateaus, visit:

http://caloriecount.about.com/new-look-weight-loss-plateaus-b425152

Don't forget that the real goal of weight loss is fat loss, so it's very helpful to keep track of your measurements in addition to monitoring your weight. If you're seeing results in your measurements and clothing sizes, then you're getting leaner even if your weight isn't dropping. That's another reason to give your body a chance to adjust to a new equilibrium before cutting calories further.

59. What do I need to know about weight loss maintenance?

Obviously, maintaining a healthy weight over a lifetime means practicing the eating and exercise habits discussed in this book. But if you've somehow been thinking of these changes as temporary, the weight-maintenance phase is the time to understand that these changes are permanent. This is the time to focus on making any mental or emotional adjustments that could stand in the way of your goals.

In an interview with WebMD, James Hill (whose work we referenced in Question 42) described weight loss as a three-stage process: weight loss, transitioning to maintenance, and maintaining the weight loss. He observed that a high level of physical activity and a good social support

To read more of the interview with Dr. Hill and find out how weight loss and weight maintenance are different, visit:

http://www.webmd.com/diet/news/20110705/tactics-are-different-for-weight loss-maintenance

system that will reinforce your lifestyle changes are both critical to successful weight loss maintenance, but also said that people tend to have trouble shifting to maintenance mode because they don't adjust their mind-set. Mental attitude—which is important to the weight loss phase—is critical to the weight-maintenance phase.

60. What will help me maintain weight loss for life?

Assuming you bring an understanding of the mechanics of healthy eating and activity to weight-maintenance mode, the three principles

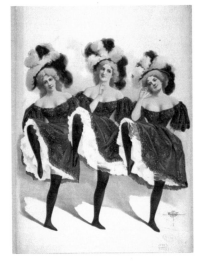

we mentioned in Question 24—transforming your sense of self, dealing with negativity, and mindfulness (awareness)—can have a big impact on whether you're able to maintain your goal weight in the long term.

Others factors—some of which we mentioned in Question 26—are also key in making lifestyle changes stick. Your reasons for making changes have to matter more to you than the status quo if they're going to help you be disciplined and persistent. And you need to get used to planning ahead if you're going to dance around obstacles as they arise.

For more advice on what it takes to lose weight for good, visit:

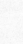

http://www.sharecare.com/question/characteristics-of-successful-weight-losers

and

http://www.sharecare.com/question/keep-off-weight-once-lost

For the difference between body-change and body-maintenance mode, visit:

http://www.builtlean.com/2012/05/09/body-change-vs-maintenance/

Be aware of your diet, your activity levels, and your weight. This may require that you stick with your tracking systems a lot longer than you hoped you'd have to, and definitely will require that you weigh yourself at least once a week. It's helpful to set your overall weight loss goal 4–5 pounds under your optimal weight to give yourself room for inevitable lapses. If you weigh yourself regularly, you'll know if you're more than three pounds above that weight, at which point it will be time to go back to tracking food and exercise very closely until you return to your starting weight. Using this approach, you'll always weigh 1–2 pounds less than your optimal weight and won't need to panic if you gain a pound or so because of water-weight gain, bad eating, skipping exercise, etc.

You need to understand that the body is programmed to fight weight loss, and that this will be a bigger problem for people who are very heavy to begin with, and probably for women (see Questions 30 and 42). When your percentage of body fat drops, the level of grehlin (the hunger hormone) increases while the levels of leptin and peptide YY (which act to suppress hunger signals) decrease (see Question 11 and Part Two Note 4). A new study shows this effect lingers well after dieting stops.

To read more about these two studies, visit:

http://www.nytimes.com/2012/01/01/magazine/tara-parker-pope-fat-trap.html?pagewanted=all&_r=0

Other research into whether leptin injections can counteract this effect is promising, but still in its very early stages.

Do what you have to manage stress, anxiety, and other emotional issues—unchecked, they're likely to sabotage you. A large body of research relates stress to overeating, insulin resistance, and general obesity. Exercise and keep your overall activity level high—it will help you manage negative emotions and also is an essential component of weight management. Change the components of your exercise routine on a regular basis. Practicing mindfulness also can help to reduce stress, and, in the process, even body fat.

For a look at the role stress plays in weight gain and metabolic issues, and the results of a study on reducing stress through practicing mindfulness, visit:

http://www.uctv.tv/shows/The-Skinny-on-Obesity-Ep-6-A-Fast-Paced-Fast-Food-Life-23721

Drink lots of water—your body needs it to do its work and it helps with weight loss and weight maintenance. Drinking a couple of glasses of water before you eat, and substituting water for another beverage, will help you stay within your calorie budget.

For the results of a study showing how drinking water helps weight loss, visit:

http://www.sciencedaily.com/releases/2010/08/100823142929.htm

For some of the research on the role sleep plays in weight management, visit:

http://www.huffingtonpost.com/2012/09/17/sleep-weight loss_n_1891171.html

Try to get enough sleep. A large body of research links prolonged sleep deprivation to a number of health problems, including obesity.

Above all, be kind to yourself.

To see the rest of the episodes in UCTV Prime's *The Skinny on Obesity* series, visit:

http://www.uctv.tv/skinny-on-obesity/

To watch HBO's *The Weight of the Nation* series, visit:

http://theweightofthenation.hbo.com/

Part Two Unlabeled Figures

Chapter 4

Part Two opening figure (left) and opening figure for chapters. Photograph of Romanesque capital (2010) courtesy of Marc Auer, available online at http://www.flickr.com/photos/pepeciseaux/4567165495

Part Two opening figure (right) and Question 21. "Get Fat On Lorings Fat-Ten-U and Corpula Foods" advertisement (ca. 1895), Library of Congress, available online at http://www.loc.gov/pictures/resource/ppmsca.05583/

Question 18. Undated photograph of morbidly obese fat child on scale crying by Jaimie Duplass, available online at http://www.shutterstock.com/cat.mhtml?lang=en&search_source=search_form&version=llv1&anyorall=all&safesearch=1&searchterm=fat+children&search_group=&orient=&search_cat=&searchtermx=&photographer_name=&people_gender=&people_age=&people_ethnicity=&people_number=&commercial_ok=&color=&show_color_wheel=1#id=79818607&src=346b6cd0a94b925ae9a27504e122c133-1-0

Question 20. Federal Art Project, WPA, "The Job of Being a Parent" poster (between 1936 and 1939), Library of Congress, available online at http://www.loc.gov/pictures/item/98517928/

Chapter 5

Question 24. Hiroshige Andō, *Zōjōji tō akabane* [Zōjōji pagoda and Akabane] (1857), Library of Congress, available online at http://www.loc.gov/pictures/collection/jpd/item/2009631887/

Question 25. Auguste Renoir, *Young Woman Braiding Her Hair* (1876), National Gallery of Art, available online at https://images.nga.gov/en/search/do_advanced_search.html?form_name=default&all_words=&exact_phrase=&exclude_words=&artist_last_name=renoir&keywords_in_title=&accession_number=&school=&Classification=&medium=&year=&year2=

Question 25. Gilbert Stuart, *The Skater (Portrait of William Grant)* (1782), National Gallery of Art, available online at https://images.nga.gov/en/set/show_content_page.html?category=16&set=17

Question 26. Photograph of potato chips courtesy of Evan-Amos (2010), available online at http://commons.wikimedia.org/wiki/File:Potato-Chips.jpg

Chapter 6

Question 30 (first figure). Undated photograph of desktop calendar by Bill Dayone, available online at http://www.shutterstock. com/cat.mhtml?lang=en&search_source=search_form&version =llv1&anyorall=all&safesearch=1&searchterm=calendar&sear ch_group=&orient=&search_cat=&searchtermx=&photographer_ name=&people_gender=&people_age=&people_ethnicity=&people_ number=&commercial_ok=&color=&show_color_ wheel=1#id=111683282

Question 30 (second figure). Undated photograph of the same girl, fat and slim by Ieva Geneviciene, available online at http://www.shutterstock.com/cat.mhtml?lang=en&search_ source=search_form&version=llv1&anyorall=all&safesea rch=1&searchterm=losing+weight+before+after&search_ group=&orient=&search_cat=&searchtermx=&photographer_ name=&people_gender=&people_age=&people_ethnicity=&people_ number=&commercial_ok=&color=&show_color_wheel=1#id=8748910

Question 35. Undated photograph of plates of food with flowers by Peggy Greb, Agricultural Research Service, USDA, available online at http://www.ars.usda.gov/is/graphics/photos/nov03/k9315-1.htm

Question 40. New York City WPA War Services, "Eat These Every Day" poster (between 1941 and 1943), Library of Congress, available online at http://www.loc.gov/pictures/item/98518333/

Chapter 7

Question 42 (first figure). Undated photograph of a healthy woman with vegetables and dumbbells by Warren Goldswain, available online at http://www.shutterstock.com/cat.mhtml?searchterm=eatin g+and+exercising&search_group=&lang=en&search_source=search_ form#id=100258688

Question 42 (second figure). Undated photograph of a tribal cave rock painting by Olga Manukyan, available online at http://www.shutterstock.com/cat.mhtml?lang=en&search_ source=search_form&version=llv1&anyorall=all&safesear ch=1&searchterm=caveman&photos=on&vectors=on&sear ch_group=&orient=&search_cat=&searchtermx=&photographer_- name=&people_gender=&people_age=&people_ethnicity=&people_ number=&commercial_ok=&color=&show_color_wheel=1&secondary_ submit=Search#id=117892804

Question 43. Hokosai Katsushika, *Sakadaru o sashiageru otoko* [Man lifting a sake barrel] (between 1804 and 1818), Library of Congress, available online at http://www.loc.gov/pictures/ item/2009615559/

Question 44. Undated photograph of a man jumping rope by Stephen Ausmus, Agricultural Research Service, USDA, available online at http://www.ars.usda.gov/is/graphics/photos/apr03/k10355-2.htm

Question 48. Undated photograph of apples by Scott Bauer, Agricultural Research Service, USDA, available online at http://www.ars.usda.gov/is/graphics/photos/k7252-65.htm

Chapter 8

Question 53. Undated photograph of pill capsules on a plate with fork and knife from Africa Studio, available online at http://www.shutterstock.com/cat.mhtml?lang=en&search_source=search_form&version=llv1&anyorall=all&safesearch=1&searchterm=weight-loss+pills&search_group=&orient=&search_cat=&searchtermx=&photographer_name=&people_gender=&people_age=&people_ethnicity=&people_number=&commercial_ok=&color=&show_color_wheel=1#id=118914193

Chapter 10

Question 58 (first figure). Carol Highsmith, photograph of Monument Valley, a Navajo Nation tribal park whose red-sandstone formations on the Colorado Plateau lie mostly in Arizona but also into Utah (between 1980 and 2006), Library of Congress, available online at http://www.loc.gov/pictures/collection/highsm/item/2011634035/

Question 58 (second figure). Strobridge Lithograph Co., *Sandow Trocadero Vaudevilles* (ca. 1894), Library of Congress, available online at http://www.loc.gov/pictures/item/var1993000227/PP/

Question 60. Courier Lithograph Co., Three dancing women in red costumes and feathers (ca. 1899), Library of Congress, available online at http://www.loc.gov/pictures/item/var1993000340/PP/

Part Two Additional Source Information

Chapter 9

Figure 9.1. Undated diagram by Alila Sao Mai, available online at http://www.shutterstock.com/cat.mhtml?searchterm=lap+banding&search_group=&lang=en&search_source=search_form#id=93594229&src=ea94cf6ce8b619932f7a0b5483c49307-1-0

Figure 9.2. Undated diagram by Alila Sao Mai, available online at http://www.shutterstock.com/cat.mhtml?lang=en&search_source=search_form&version=llv1&anyorall=all&safesearch=1&searchterm=Roux-en-Y+gastric+bypass&search_group=&orient=&search_cat=&searchtermx=&photographer_name=&people_gender=&people_age=&people_ethnicity=&people_number=&commercial_ok=&color=&show_color_wheel=1#id=93594220&src=665393c78bbdffee98d280fd8c7de76e-1-1

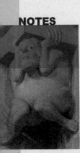

Figure 9.3. Undated diagram by Alila Sao Mai, available online at http://www.shutterstock.com/cat.mhtml?searchterm=Vertical+sleev e+gastrectomy&search_group=&lang=en&search_source=search_fo rm#id=93594679&src=9155a3b4a604e2286de7dcb9e783f90c-1-0

Part Two Notes

REFERENCE

Chapter 4

1. Although the U.S. Preventative Services Task Force (USPSTF) has recommended screening children age six and older for overweight and obesity, the American Academy of Pediatrics continues to recommend universal screening. See Sandra G. Hassink, "Evidence for Effective Obesity Treatment: Pediatricians on the Right Track!", *Pediatrics* 125:2 (2010), 387–388, available online at http://pediatrics.aappublications.org/content/125/2/387. full.pdf, September 25, 2012.

2. National Heart, Lung, and Blood Institute (NHLBI), NIH, *Working Group Report on Future Research Directions in Childhood Obesity Prevention and Treatment* (2007), available online at http://www.nhlbi.nih.gov/meetings/workshops/child-obesity/index.htm, September 26, 2012.

3. See Harrison Wein, "Where Kids Get Their Empty Calories," NIH Research Matters (October 25, 2010), available online at http://www.nih.gov/researchmatters/october2010/10252010empty calories.htm, September 26, 2012.

Chapter 5

4. Ghrelin is a hormone in the stomach that's responsible for telling the brain that you're hungry. The level of ghrelin rises before you eat and falls after you eat, but it's not the hormone that tells the brain you're full. For the brain to get that signal, the food must first move through the twenty-two feet of the intestine via peristalsis (the waves of contraction that push the food along). Cells at the end of the intestine release a hormone called peptide YY, which sends a signal to the brain that the body has reached a state of satiety, or fullness. This process takes about twenty minutes, although the brain gets the signal a few minutes quicker if dietary fiber—which helps move food along in the intestine—is consumed as part of the meal.

5. Anyone who has lost at least 30 pounds and kept it off for at least a year can join the NWCR. Currently the NWCR is tracking over 10,000 individuals who fill out detailed questionnaires and annual surveys to help it with its mission. See the NWCR Web site at http://www.nwcr.ws/default.htm

6. G. A. Marlatt and J. L. Kristeller, "Mindfulness and Meditation." In W. R. Miller (ed.), *Integrating Spirituality into Treatment* (Washington, D.C.: American Psychological Association, 1999), 67–84.

7. See "He Shed, She Shed: Herbalife Surveys How Men And Women View Weight Loss," Medical News Today (January 9, 2011), available online at http://www.medicalnewstoday.com/articles/213102.php, October 10, 2012.

8. See WeightWatchers Research Department, "Gender Differences in Motivators and Barriers to Weight Loss," WeightWatchers (November 12, 2012), available online at http://www.weightwatchers.com/util/art/index_art.aspx?tabnum=1&art_id=35491&sc=802#footnotes, November 20, 2012.

9. See Document 6.16.AimHthyWgt on the DVD.

Chapter 6

10. Basal metabolic rate (BMR) is a precise measurement of basic calorie requirements and is typically performed in a test facility. The measurement is taken with the subject reclining in a darkened room after eight hours of sleep and twelve hours of fasting (the latter in order to exclude energy requirements for digestive activities). Resting metabolic rate (RMR) usually is measured under less restrictive conditions and often includes calories devoted to digestion. The term BMR (also known as **basal energy expenditure**, or **BEE**) frequently is used synonymously with—and may be more readily recognized than—RMR (also known as **resting energy expenditure**, or **REE**) and hence the two terms are used interchangeably throughout this book.

11. All Question 27 calorie expenditure percentages from Mayo Clinic, "Metabolism and Weight Loss: How You Burn Calories," available online at http://www.mayoclinic.com/health/metabolism/WT00006, October 10, 2012.

12. Alexandra M. Johnstone et al., "Factors Influencing Variation in Basal Metabolic Rate Include Fat-Free Mass, Fat Mass, Age, and Circulating Thyroxine but Not Sex, Circulating Leptin, or Triiodothyronine," *American Journal of Clinical Nutrition* 82:5 (2005), 941–948, available online at http://ajcn.nutrition.org/content/82/5/941.abstract, October 10, 2012.

13. There are three types of **thermogenesis** (the process of heat production in the body): **exercise-associated thermogenesis (EAT), non-exercise activity thermogenesis (NEAT), and diet-induced thermogenesis (DIT)**. EAT is heat production through exercise, NEAT is heat production through spontaneous physical activity (routine, low-intensity activities, such as fidgeting or scratching your ear), and DIT is heat production through the ingestion of food.

14. See Marion Nestle's August 4, 2011 interview with the *Atlantic*, available online at http://www.theatlantic.com/health/archive/2011/08/why-does-the-fda-recommend-2-000-calories-per-day/243092/, November 19, 2012.

15. American College of Sports Medicine, "Metabolism is Modifiable with the Right Lifestyle Changes," available online at http://www.acsm.org/about-acsm/media-room/acsm-in-the-news/2011/08/01/metabolism-is-modifiable-with-the-right-lifestyle-changes, November 9, 2012.

16. For this quotation and other information referenced in Question 30 (unless cited otherwise), see Kevin D. Hall et al., "Quantification of the Effect of Energy Imbalance on Bodyweight," *Lancet* 378:9793 (2011), 826–37, available online at http://www.thelancet.com/journals/lancet/article/PIIS0140-6736(11)60812-x/fulltext, November 9, 2012.

17. D. A. Schoeller and C. R. Fjeld, "Human Energy Metabolism: What Have We Learned from the Doubly Labeled Water Method?", *Annual Review of Nutrition* 11:1 (1991), 355–73.

18. Food and Drug Administration (FDA), "Appendix F: Calculate the Percent Daily Value for the Appropriate Nutrients," in *Guidance for Industry: A Food Labeling Guide*, available online at http://www.fda.gov/Food/GuidanceComplianceRegulatoryInformation/GuidanceDocuments/FoodLabelingNutrition/FoodLabelingGuide/ucm064928.htm, November 30, 2012.

19. Andrea Carlson and Elizabeth Frazao, *Are Healthy Foods Really More Expensive? It Depends on How You Measure the Price*, U.S. Department of Agriculture, Economic Research Service, available online at http://www.ers.usda.gov/publications/eib-economic-information-bulletin/eib96.aspx, November 30, 2012.

20. United Press International, "Americans Eat Out About Five Times a Week," available online at http://www.upi.com/Health_News/2011/09/19/Americans-eat-out-about-5-times-a-week/UPI-54241316490172/, November 30, 2012.

Chapter 7

21. James O. Hill and Holly R. Wyatt, "Role of Physical Activity in Preventing and Treating Obesity," *Journal of Applied Physiology* 99:2 (2005), 765, available online at http://www.jappl.org/content/99/2/765.full, November 1, 2012.

22. Jean Mayer, Purnima Roy, and Kamakhya Prasad Mitra, "Relation between Calorie Intake, Body Weight, and Physical Work: Studies in an Industrial Male Population in West Bengal," *American Journal of Clinical Nutrition* 4:2 (1956), 174, available online at http://ajcn.nutrition.org/content/4/2/169.full.pdf+html, November 3, 2012.

23. Mary L. Johnson, Bertha S. Burke, and Jean Mayer, "Relative Importance of Inactivity and Overeating in the Energy Balance of Obese High School Girls," *American Journal of Clinical Nutrition* 4:1 (1956), 37–44, available online at http://ajcn.nutrition.org/content/4/1/37.full.pdf+html, November 3, 2012.

24. D. A. Schoeller, "Balancing Energy Expenditure and Body Weight," *American Journal of Clinical Nutrition* 68:4 (1998), 956S, available online at http://ajcn.nutrition.org/content/68/4/956S.full.pdf+html, November 3, 2012.

25. Jean Mayer, Purnima Roy, and Kamakhya Prasad Mitra, "Relation between Calorie Intake, Body Weight, and Physical Work: Studies in an Industrial Male Population in West Bengal," *American Journal of Clinical Nutrition* 4:2 (1956), 174, available online at http://ajcn.nutrition.org/content/4/2/169.full.pdf+html, November 3, 2012.

26. James O. Hill, Holly R. Wyatt, and John C. Peters, "Energy Balance and Obesity," *Circulation* 126:1 (2012), 126, available online at http://www.ucdenver.edu/about/newsroom/newsreleases/PublishingImages/2012-07/Hill_Circulation.pdf, November 3, 2012.

27. Ibid, 127.

28. U.S. Department of Health and Human Services, *Physical Activity Guidelines for Americans* (2008), vii–viii (see Document 7.1.PAGuide).

29. From Kate Ridley, Barbara Ainsworth, and Tim Olds, "Development of a Compendium of Energy Expenditures for Youth," *International Journal of Behavioral Nutrition and Physical Activity* 5:45 (2008), available online at http://www.ijbnpa.org/content/5/1/45, January 14, 2013.

30. Harvard Health Publications, "Calories Burned in 30 Minutes for People of Three Different Weights," available online at http://www.health.harvard.edu/newsweek/Calories-burned-in-30-minutes-of-leisure-and-routine-activities.htm, January 18, 2013.

31. See the Obesity Prevention Source, Harvard School of Public Health, "Television Watching and 'Sit Time,'" available online at http://www.hsph.harvard.edu/obesity-prevention-source/obesity-causes/television-and-sedentary-behavior-and-obesity/, January 18, 2013.

32. Steven L. Gortmaker et al., "Television Viewing as a Cause of Increasing Obesity among Children in the United States, 1986–1990," *Archives of Pediatrics and Adolescent Medicine* 150:4 (1996), abstract available online at http://www.ncbi.nlm.nih.gov/pubmed/8634729, January 18, 2013.

Chapter 8

33. Trivalent chromium, which is thought to be benign, should not be confused with hexavalent chromium, or chromium 6+, a toxic industrial by-product.

34. Joe A. Vinson, Bryan R. Burnham, and Mysore V. Nagendran, "Randomized, Double-Blind, Placebo-Controlled, Linear Dose, Crossover Study to Evaluate the Efficacy and Safety of a Green Coffee Bean Extract in Overweight Subjects," *Diabetes, Metabolic Syndrome, and Obesity: Targets and Therapy* 5 (2012), 21–27, available online at http://www.worldcat.org/title/randomized-double-blind-placebo-controlled-linear-dose-crossover-study-to-evaluate-the-efficacy-and-safety-of-a-green-coffee-bean-extract-in-overweight-subjects/oclc/776189836&referer=brief_results, January 18, 2013.

35. Chromium picolinate is a chemical compound made from trivalent chromium and picolinic acid.

Chapter 10

36. On research comparing the metabolic rates of obese and nonobese individuals, see Roland L. Weinsier et al., "Do Adaptive Changes in Metabolic Rate Favor Weight Regain in Weight-Reduced Individuals? An Examination of the Set-Point Theory," *American Journal of Clinical Nutrition* 72:5 (2000), 1088–1094, available online at http://ajcn.nutrition.org/content/72/5/1088.full, January 24, 2013. (For a discussion of the research results see Victoria Stagg Elliott, "Research Challenges Theory That Weight Has a Set Point," *American Medical News* (February 12, 2001), available online at http://www.ama-assn.org/amednews/2001/02/12/hlsc0212.htm, January 24, 2013.)

On bariatric surgery resulting in a new set point, see M. M. Farias, A. M. Cuevas, and F. Rodriguez, "Set-Point Theory and Obesity," *Metabolic Syndrome and Related Disorders* 9:2 (2011), 85–89, abstract available online at http://www.ncbi.nlm.nih.gov/pubmed/21117971, January 24, 2013.

Index

20-minute rule, 46

A

abdominal fat, 6
absolute intensity, 79–80
acai berry, 94
active children, 86–87
Adipex-P®, 88
adipose tissue, 4
adjustable gastric banding (AGB),
    98
adult body-fat range, 9
adults
    exercise for, 77
    health care professionals, 38–39
aerobic activity, 74
AGB. *See* adjustable gastric banding
Alli®, 91
AMA. *See* American Medical
    Association
Amazonian palm berry, 94
American Academy of Pediatrics, 86
American College of Sports Medicine,
    57
American Medical Association
    (AMA), 40, 98
android obesity, 9
anesthesiologists, 29–30
anesthetic health risk, 29–30
anticonvulsant drug. *See* topiramate
appetite, 44
apple-shaped body, 9
atheromatous plaque deposits, 23
atherosclerosis, 23
attitude, 107

B

bad cholesterol, 21
balance activity, 75–76
bariatric surgery
    adjustable gastric banding, 98
    biliopancreatic diversion with
        duodenal switch, 99–100
    considerations, 96–97
    Roux-en-Y gastric bypass surgery,
        98–99
    vertical sleeve gastrectomy, 99
basal metabolic rate (BMR), 53–55
belly fat, 6
Belviq®, 92

BIA. *See* bioelectrical impedance
    analysis
biliopancreatic diversion (BPD), 99
biliopancreatic diversion with
    duodenal switch (BPD-DS),
    99–100
biliopancreatic loop, 100
bioelectrical impedance analysis
    (BIA), 7
bitter orange, 94–95
blood lipids, 21
blood pressure (BP), 25–26
BMI. *See* body mass index
BMR. *See* basal metabolic rate
Body Benchmark Study, 8
body-fat monitors, 7
body fat, normal percentage, 8–9
body-fat scales, 7
body frame, 6
body mass index (BMI)
    calculation, 5–6
    categories, 4–5
    definition, 4
    drug treatment for obesity, 88
body volume index (BVI), 8
bone-strengthening activity, 74–75
bottlefeeding *vs.* breastfeeding,
    14–15
BP. *See* blood pressure
BPD. *See* biliopancreatic diversion
BPD-DS. *See* biliopancreatic
    diversion with duodenal
    switch
breastfed infants, 15
bupropion, 93
BVI. *See* body volume index

C

calipers, 7
calorie
    activities burn, 80–81
    for current weight, 54–57
    definition, 10
    information, 67
    tips for reduction, 67–68
cancer-related risk, 30–31
cardiovascular activity. *See* aerobic
    activity
CDC. *See* Centers for Disease
    Control and Prevention

NHBLI. *See* National Heart, Blood, and Lung Institute
NIDD. *See* non-insulin dependent diabetes
non-insulin dependent diabetes (NIDD), 26
nutrition
  childhood obesity
    early, 15–16
    during pregnancy, 14
  information, 67
  labels, 63–64
NWCR. *See* National Weight Control Registry

O

obesity
  android, 9
  causes of, 10
  childhood, 13–20
  definition, 4
  drug treatment, 88–93
  gynoid, 9
  health risks, 21–30
  herbal supplements, 93–96
  hyperplastic, 15–16
  hypertrophic, 15–16
  other factors, 10–11
  prevalence, 11
  psychological effects, 31
  social effects, 31
  surgical treatment, 96–100
obesity treatment
  health care professionals
    adults, 38–39
    children, 39–41
    parents role, 42–43
    patients role, 41–42
    strategies, 43
    weight-management program, 43–44
obstructive sleep apnea (OSA), 28–29
off-label use, 88
older adults, exercise, 77
open surgery, 97
orlistat, 91–92
OSA. *See* obstructive sleep apnea
osteoarthritis, 27
ovulation, 28

P

PCOS. *See* polycystic ovary syndrome
pear-shaped body, 9
phentermine, 88–89
phentermine-topiramate, 90–91
physical activity
  aerobic activity, 74
  balance activity, 75–76
  bone-strengthening activity, 74–75
  vs. exercise, 71–72
  muscle-strengthening activity, 74–75
  routine, 71
  stretching, 75
  weight control, 72–74
  weight loss plateaus, 105–107
physical fitness, 71
plateaus, 101
polycystic ovary syndrome (PCOS), 28
portion, 63
preeclampsia, 28
pregnancy
  exercise during, 78
  health risk problems, 28
  nutrition during, 14
pyloric valve, 99

Q

Qsymia™, 90

R

RDIs. *See* reference daily intakes
reference daily intakes (RDIs), 65
relative intensity, 80
resting metabolic rate (RMR), 53
restrictive bariatric surgery, 97
RMR. *See* resting metabolic rate
routine physical activity, 71
Roux-en-Y gastric bypass (RYGB) surgery, 98–99

S

safety, weight loss, 57
scheduling exercise, 82–84
serving size, 63
set-point theory, 101
skinfold thickness, 7
stimulant drug. *See* diethypropion
stomach stapling, 98

strength training, 74
stretching, 75
subcutaneous fat, 6
SuperTracker, 65–66
surgical treatment. *See* bariatric
    surgery

T

Tenuate®, 89
Tenuate Dospan®, 89
Topamax®, 89
topiramate, 89–90
triglycerides, 21
trivalent chromium, 95
type 1 diabetes, 26
type 2 diabetes, 26

U

U.S. Preventive Services Task Force
    (USPSTF), 41
USPSTF. *See* U.S. Preventive
    Services Task Force

V

vertical banded gastroplasty (VGB),
    98
vertical sleeve gastrectomy (VSG), 99
VGB. *See* vertical banded
    gastroplasty
vigorous-intensity activities, 79–80
visceral fat, 6
VSG. *See* vertical sleeve gastrectomy

W

waist circumference, 7
waist-to-hip ratio, 7
weight control, 72–74

weight loss
    diet, 64–66
    habits
        current status, 51
        goal definition and creating plan,
            50–51
        reasons for change, 51
        self-preparation, 52
        small and specific, 51–52
        tracking progress, 52–53
    maintenance, 107–108
    motivation, 49
    other factors, 108–110
    role of mind
        mindfulness over will power,
            48–49
        negativity, 47–48
        redefining identity, 47
        thinking style, 47
    safety measures, 57
    surgery, 96–100
weight loss plateaus
    attitude, 107
    definition, 101
    description, 101–103
    diet, 103–105
    physical activity, 105–107
weight-management program, 43–44
weight training, 74
Wellbutrin®, 93
willpower, 48–49

X

Xenical®, 91

Z

zhi shi, 94